Praise for
Staff Educator's Guide to Clinical Orientation

"This marvelous resource will positively enrich your clinical onboarding program. The book is comprehensive and harmonizes theory and practice with easy-to-implement tools. A must-have for all nursing professionals involved in new employee orientation."

−Cindy Borum, MSN, APRN, FNP-C
Assistant Vice President, HCA Healthcare

"The second edition of *Staff Educator's Guide to Clinical Orientation* provides a comprehensive yet easy-to-navigate resource to effectively onboard and orient nurses to clinical departments. The book provides guidance in establishing a new program as well as helpful advice to those needing to refresh their existing program—with both low and high technology options to meet the needs of facilities with varying levels of means. This comprehensive resource includes information for leaders, educators, and preceptors, emphasizing that onboarding is a process, not an event, and can continue well beyond the allotted orientation time. The book covers numerous aspects of the onboarding process, including the critical aspect of providing effective feedback for the orientee. It pulls from different industries, expanding the reader's global thinking outside of the healthcare industry for application of concepts. Lastly, this well-written resource provides wide-ranging examples, case studies, and lessons learned to guide the reader through the development of a clinical orientation program in these complex healthcare times."

−Vicki Good, DNP, RN, CPPS
Administrative Director Clinical Safety
CoxHealth, Springfield, Missouri

"Jeffery, Jarvis, and Word-Allen put the orientation and onboarding process into contemporary language and recognize the complexities of good onboarding in healthcare. The book is easy to read and offers real-world solutions to implementing and evaluating onboarding programs. Well done!"

−Catherine H. Ivory, PhD, RN-BC, FAAN
Associate Chief Nurse Executive, Vice President,
Professional Practice & Care Transformation
Indiana University Health
Assistant Dean for Care Transformation,
Indiana University School of Nursing

STAFF EDUCATOR'S GUIDE TO

Clinical Orientation

Second Edition

Onboarding Solutions for Nurses

Alvin D. Jeffery, PhD, RN-BC, CCRN-K, FNP-BC
Robin L. Jarvis, MS, SPHR
with **Amy J. Word-Allen, BSN, RN**

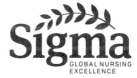

Sigma
GLOBAL NURSING
EXCELLENCE

The Sigma Theta Tau International Honor Society of Nursing (Sigma) is a nonprofit organization whose mission is advancing world health and celebrating nursing excellence in scholarship, leadership, and service. Founded in 1922, Sigma has more than 135,000 active members in over 90 countries and territories. Members include practicing nurses, instructors, researchers, policymakers, entrepreneurs, and others. Sigma's more than 530 chapters are located at more than 700 institutions of higher education throughout Armenia, Australia, Botswana, Brazil, Canada, Colombia, England, Ghana, Hong Kong, Japan, Jordan, Kenya, Lebanon, Malawi, Mexico, the Netherlands, Pakistan, Philippines, Portugal, Singapore, South Africa, South Korea, Swaziland, Sweden, Taiwan, Tanzania, Thailand, the United States, and Wales. Learn more at www.sigmanursing.org.

550 West North Street I Indianapolis, IN, USA 46202

To order additional books, buy in bulk, or order for corporate use, contact Sigma Marketplace at 888.654.4968/US and Canada or +1.317.634.8171 (outside US and Canada).

To request a review copy for course adoption, email solutions@sigmanursing.org or call 888.654.4968/US and Canada or +1.317.634.8171 (outside US and Canada).

To request author information, or for speaker or other media requests, contact Sigma Marketing at 888.634.7575 (US and Canada) or +1.317.634.8171 (outside US and Canada).

ISBN: 9781945157677   EPUB ISBN: 9781945157684
PDF ISBN: 9781945157691   MOBI ISBN: 9781945157707

Library of Congress Cataloging-in-Publication Data

Names: Jeffery, Alvin D., 1986- author. I Jarvis, Robin L., 1962- author. I Word-Allen, Amy, author. I Sigma Theta Tau International, issuing body.

Title: Staff educator's guide to clinical orientation : onboarding solutions for nurses / Alvin D. Jeffery, Robin L. Jarvis ; with Amy Word-Allen.

Description: Second edition. I Indianapolis, IN, USA : Sigma Theta Tau International, [2018] I Includes bibliographical references and index.

Identifiers: LCCN 2017054296 (print) I LCCN 2017055066 (ebook) I ISBN 9781945157684 (Epub) I ISBN 9781945157691 (Pdf) I ISBN 9781945157707 (Mobi) I ISBN 9781945157677 (print : alk. paper) I ISBN 9781945157707 (mobi)

Subjects: I MESH: Education, Nursing, Continuing I Inservice Training—methods I Inservice Training—organization & administration I Professional Competence

Classification: LCC RT76 (ebook) I LCC RT76 (print) I NLM WY 18.5 I DDC 610.73071/55—dc23

LC record available at https://lccn.loc.gov/2017054296

First Printing, 2018

Publisher: Dustin Sullivan   Principal Book Editor: Carla Hall
Acquisitions Editor: Emily Hatch   Development and Project Editor: Kezia Endsley
Editorial Coordinator: Paula Jeffers   Copy Editor: Erin Geile
Cover Designer: Michael Tanamachi   Proofreader: Todd Lothery
Interior Design/Page Layout: Michael Tanamachi   Indexer: Larry D. Sweazy

Dedications

In memory of our grandfather and father, Kenneth D. Jarvis, who taught both of us that if you could read about it, you could do something about it.
–Alvin & Robin

To my spouse, Jamey, for his love and support during the writing of this book and my many scholarly adventures. –Alvin

To the memory of my beloved wife, Susan, who supported me in all my endeavors. –Robin

To my son, Mason. You have been and always will be my sunshine. Your spirit teaches me to be young at heart and keep moving forward. I love you, bear. –Amy

Acknowledgments

Alvin would like to thank Rhonda Cooper for ensuring the accuracy and completeness of the student and academic partnership information.

Robin would like to acknowledge Debra R. France, EdD, who, with Robin, co-designed and developed SEMATECH's orientation program. Debra is a gifted learning and development professional and someone to whom Robin always will look for ideas, camaraderie, and creativity.

Amy would like to thank Robin and Alvin for helping her cultivate her very first book. She feels their expertise and faith in her skills made the project possible for her. She'd also like to thank her teachers, whose faith and hard work inspire her to be better and for seeing her potential and pushing her to it. Her tribe, for being there in moments of failure *and* celebration, for showing up to cheer her on and help her remember who she is, and for challenging her and showing her what it is like to be loved. And her family. "I am what I am because of y'all. There isn't a thing in this world that makes me less than enough for my family. Thank you for believing, fighting, showing up, sacrificing, teaching, nurturing, and loving me perfectly for me. My cup truly runneth over."

We'd also like reiterate the significant contributions from several key persons during the writing of the first edition of the book:

David D. Jarvis, for providing insights from the perspective of nursing home facilities, for making sure that things made sense, and for being a great uncle and brother!

Bill Jeffery, for offering guidance on the flow of content, for providing some humorous remarks, and for being a great nephew and brother!

Dena Clark and Beth Mueller, for making sure Alvin stayed on topic but also included all the important information for educators. Dena and Beth are two of the most remarkable nurse educators, colleagues, and friends, and Alvin loved every day he was able to work with them.

About the Authors

Alvin D. Jeffery, PhD, RN-BC, CCRN-K, FNP-BC

Alvin D. Jeffery is a recent PhD graduate from Vanderbilt University in Nashville, Tennessee. He is currently employed as a research fellow with the U.S. Department of Veterans Affairs, where he studies nursing-focused informatics interventions. He currently holds part-time appointments as an Education Consultant at Cincinnati Children's Hospital Medical Center in Cincinnati, Ohio, and as a Nurse Scientist with the Hospital Corporation of America in Nashville, Tennessee.

Before pursuing his PhD, Jeffery worked as the unit-based educator in a pediatric intensive care unit at Cincinnati Children's Hospital Medical Center. During this time as an educator, Jeffery finished his master of science in nursing (MSN) degree with a focus as a family nurse practitioner (FNP). He is board-certified in both Nursing Professional Development (American Nurses Credentialing Center) and Pediatric Critical-Care Nursing (American Association of Critical-Care Nurses), and he has developed and instructed internal review courses for both of these certifications.

Jeffery has facilitated several internal inservices/continuing education programs in various aspects of nursing professional and staff development and has served as a preceptor for several new educators in the pediatric intensive care unit. He has collaborated with almost every department to help organize, design, and develop various staff development projects including, but not limited to, competency assessment tools, education record management databases, simulation implementation, and preceptor development. He is one of the authors of this book's first edition as well as the *Staff Educator's Guide to Professional Development*.

Robin L. Jarvis, MS, SPHR

Robin L. Jarvis is an expert in adult learning with over 25 years of experience in high technology, retail, and consulting companies. She has experience in leadership development, talent management, and organizational development, as well as serving as an HR generalist and leading a talent-acquisition team. Her work has taken her from Texas to India, China, Singapore, Taiwan, and England.

In addition to a master of science in leadership, Jarvis has participated in over 500 hours of additional training in topics such as cross-cultural communication, accelerated learning, instructional design, leadership development, brain-based learning, neuro-linguistic programming, and meeting and workshop facilitation. She has designed and delivered workshops on topics including new employee orientation and onboarding, change management, employee engagement, career development, accelerated learning, learning styles, Myers-Briggs Type Indicator (MBTI), StrengthsFinder, *The 7 Habits of Highly Effective People*, presentation skills, meeting skills, behavioral-based interviewing, and many other topics.

Jarvis has co-presented at several conferences on the topic of orientation and onboarding. She and Debra R. France, EdD, co-authored an article, "Quick Starts for New Employees," which was published in *Training and Development* magazine. She and France received SEMATECH's corporate award for the orientation program they designed.

Amy J. Word-Allen, BSN, RN

Amy J. Word-Allen is currently employed with Avalon Hospice. She has 2 years of burn center experience with pediatric and adult patients. She worked in the pediatric critical care unit at Monroe Carell Jr. Children's Hospital at Vanderbilt, where she served as a clinical staff nurse, primary preceptor, unit board president, primary/secondary preceptor, charge nurse, interim assistant manager, and on the education committee. She worked in onboarding roles, serving on the board interviewing pediatric nursing residents, interviewing experienced staff nurses, conducting peer interviews, and developing didactic classroom orientation content. She also developed guidelines for primary preceptors and presentations for educators to utilize during orientation.

Word-Allen has worked as adjunct faculty for Tennessee Tech University as the pediatric clinical professor and in the pediatric ICU at the Children's Hospital at TriStar Centennial in Nashville, Tennessee, where she served as lead preceptor/mentor, developed the clinical orientation for the PICU with managers, and served as a charge nurse. She developed teaching materials and presented in the skills fair for the continuing education of all the pediatric nurses within the organization. She built a mentoring program to pair orientees with coworkers to provide support during the first year of employment. During her time as a lead preceptor, she also served as one of four primary preceptors on the unit. She has facilitated multiple orientation experiences for staff nurses and has developed strategies to help preceptors teach and connect deeper to their orientees. She has worked in multiple roles in the process of precepting and mentoring. She has spent over 3,250 hours precepting staff.

Table of Contents

Introduction to the Second Edition

Welcome to the second edition of the *Staff Educator's Guide to Clinical Orientation*! We are so excited that we have this opportunity to improve and expand on the content from the first edition!

In speaking with staff educators and preceptors about the book over the last few years, we've heard amazing stories of nurses overcoming orientation challenges through their innovation, creativity, and unending passion for training new employees. Since publishing the first edition in 2014, many aspects of the nursing landscape have remained unchanged: Turnover and satisfaction remain problematic, schools are still producing new graduate nurses, and organizations are asking that we reduce the length of orientation. But a few things are changing: Patients are getting sicker, payments for healthcare services in the US are becoming more complex, and technology is playing a larger role in healthcare delivery.

Admittedly, we are a bit biased, but we believe the nursing professional development specialist (that is, the staff educator) is well-poised to help address these challenges. Staff educators are leaders within the organization who are sufficiently skilled (and trusted!) to communicate directly with C-suite leaders and direct care clinicians. The opportunities for staff educators to develop a nursing and healthcare workforce that can address current and future barriers to optimal care are plentiful! Although it's not the end of the story, a significant portion of this work begins with orientation and onboarding programs.

A high-functioning orientation program is essential to delivering high-quality care. But a good program doesn't happen overnight, or all by itself. Developing and sustaining a great onboarding program requires time, commitment, critiques, and constant evolution. And that's exactly what we want to help you with!

The *Staff Educator's Guide to Clinical Orientation* covers conceptual and practical advice for all aspects of orientating and onboarding nurses. Of course, the content could be applied to several other healthcare and non-healthcare professionals, but all of our examples are nursing-centric. In this second edition, we have added several new resources, updated the references (when available), and included a whole new chapter focused on students and contract employees. Much of the flow and content, however, has remained unchanged because readers have expressed they've found it helpful.

We'll begin with an overview of the more conceptual pieces of orientation and introduce the ADDIE model for instructional design. We include examples, tables, and worksheets to help you apply the principles immediately. We become more concrete as we move into a discussion of implementing the various facets of an orientation program, and we spend some time providing tips and tricks for a wide variety of orientee types and challenges. We finish the book with some thoughts on regulatory and legal issues as well as several resources for staying organized.

In addition to the new chapter and updated resources, we've also added a new voice in the book—the preceptor. The role of the preceptor cannot be overstated in orientation activities, and in some organizations where there is not a formal staff educator to oversee education, preceptors might be responsible for most of the orientation and onboarding activities. To provide this perspective, we have invited Amy Word-Allen to write preceptor and mentor-focused content for us.

Alvin's most recent clinical position was in a 10-bed pediatric ICU at a community hospital, and Amy was his preceptor for orientation. Amy recounts, "I crossed paths with Alvin in 2015. I had assumed my primary preceptor role and had developed what I felt was a comprehensive program, but like any new task or skill, you are always unsure of how implementation will look.

"Our unit-based orientation was small enough that I could take on the task of orienting new staff. When I saw Alvin's résumé, I knew he would be mine. The other preceptors were younger and finding their solid footing, so they didn't need the super educated to come in and ask the 'Why?' question so much they didn't feel successful. And by all of my assessments, Alvin was going to be smart, he was going to know what he was doing, and he would be able to recite research like the back of his hand.

"I was skeptical the first day. He was perky, motivated, ready to dive into practical care, and highly knowledgeable of the 'how.' My job was to dig into the 'why' and let his muscle memory have time to kick back in. I dreaded it because I knew he was going to know more than me, but it was evident that not only could I have a skill set to teach him, but he was enthusiastic about being in touch with the practical side of nursing.

"We ended up being a great pair. Our time flowed together, and he was really ready to not only share his knowledge in a nonjudgmental way but also glean knowledge of the practical side of nursing. We shared meals, we laughed, we cried, we shared frustrations of our professional careers, and we discussed how to make him better. I felt really good about letting him out into the unit to practice by the end of our time together."

We're excited to expand the book's audience to be a bit more inclusive of preceptors with the addition of Amy's "Preceptor Pointers."

We hope you'll find the book an engaging read with helpful advice on creating and maintaining a high-quality orientation and onboarding program. We have enjoyed creating the content for you, and we wish you success in all your teaching and mentoring efforts!

Foreword

I have often referred to the first few days of orientation as a "parade of stars." For several days, a parade of experts from across the organization tell new employees all about their own role, touching very little on useful information that will help newcomers learn their jobs. The cumulative impact of this approach is often a bewildered and confused new nurse. The second edition of *Staff Educator's Guide to Clinical Orientation* provides educators and leaders with the antidote to this very common ailment in nurse orientation and onboarding programs.

I have experienced the parade of stars approach to orientation as a nurse, preceptor, educator, and leader. Now, as the Chief Nurse Executive of a large healthcare system, I am on a mission to obliterate it. This book offers meaningful alternatives and practical tools for how to design and implement an effective orientation and onboarding approach that engages and supports new nurses starting with their first day.

I've had the pleasure of working with Alvin Jeffery when he was a doctoral student and more recently as a nurse scientist. This book is grounded in evidence, as you would expect from a nurse scientist, but also has practical tools and real-world case examples provided by all the authors. Amy Word-Allen's focus on preceptors is a welcome addition to the second edition.

Robin Jarvis and Alvin Jeffery have structured the entire book as an illustration of adult learning principles. They alternate theory and application throughout the book. Each chapter concludes with questions for reflection and key takeaways. Chapters on temporary staff and regulatory compliance reflect their awareness of the day-to-day challenges of nurse educators.

So, join the movement! Let's replace the parade of stars with meaningful orientation and onboarding programs that engage and support nurses from the first day of employment. This book shows us how to do it.

–Jane Englebright, PhD, RN, CENP, FAAN
Senior Vice President & Chief Nurse Executive
HCA | Clinical Services Group

Introduction

"I never teach my pupils; I only attempt to provide the conditions in which they can learn." –Albert Einstein

Welcome to the *Staff Educator's Guide to Clinical Orientation*! Throughout this book, we want to provide you with tools and techniques for creating and sustaining those ideal conditions to which Einstein refers. We hope you'll find this book an enjoyable and insightful discussion of how to develop orientation and onboarding programs for nurses that will result in well-prepared orientees and satisfied organizational stakeholders.

Our goal in writing this book is to provide you with a quick reference or just-in-time field guide to making your orientation programs successful. We know that you have a busy schedule, so we have included several worksheets and tools that can be used immediately in case you don't have the time to read a more lengthy discussion on a particular topic. We hope you will read the entire book so that you can understand the tools and adapt them more to your individual needs, but we wanted to give you something you could use *today*.

We have written this text for nursing professional development specialists (that is, nurse educators in the clinical setting) as well as managers and administrators who work with nurses in orientation. Although preceptors and senior-level administrators may learn new concepts from these readings, the intended audience includes those mid-level leaders who dabble in day-to-day orientation/onboarding activities as well as the design, development, and implementation of orientation/onboarding programs. Our experience has shown that many mid-level leaders are not fully equipped in formal training and development concepts that are essential to effective and efficient orientation/onboarding programs. This book is intended to help bridge this knowledge gap.

Because we want you to use this as a field guide, we are providing an overview of each chapter so that you know where to go for your specific issue or concern. Each chapter has some suggested reflection/discussion questions for you to consider. We hope that you find these questions as well as the worksheets, tables, etc., helpful.

Chapter 1
Important Considerations for Onboarding and Orientation

This chapter provides you with an overview of the ADDIE model (Analyze, Design, Develop, Implement, and Evaluate), which is the standard model for designing training programs such as onboarding and orientation. You might notice the similarities between the ADDIE model and one you use every day in nursing (Assess, Diagnose, Plan, Implement, and Evaluate).

The ADDIE model really provides the basis for the rest of the book. We look at each step in the model throughout the book. The remainder of Chapter 1 looks at principles and principals for your program. Principles are key things to consider during the development of your program. The principals are all the stakeholders in this important program and process.

Chapter 2
Analysis and Design of an Onboarding Program

Chapter 2 looks at the first two steps in the ADDIE model—Analyze and Design. In the Analyze step, we address a few data-gathering modes and even provide a focus-group agenda for you to use. If you have an existing program, we provide some tips on how to assess the strengths and weaknesses of your program, as well as point out some errors to avoid. If you're creating a new program, this chapter will give you the tools you need to get started by ensuring you know what your organization needs.

During the Analyze step, you must understand your learners, so we talk about some models that address how people learn. We limit it to three models, as we believe that the application of these three will ensure that your learners' needs are met. Many of you are familiar with the American Association of Critical-Care Nurses (AACN) Synergy Model, and we discuss how that can be applied to your analysis and design. We also discuss making recommendations to key stakeholders when you have finished the Analyze phase, and we provide some worksheets and examples to get you started with the Design phase.

Chapter 3
Developing and Implementing an Orientation Program

This chapter takes the design worksheets we introduced in Chapter 2 and guides you on how to use those to develop your orientation and onboarding modules. We provide examples at the organizational and unit level, just as we did in Chapter 2. We also include examples of facilitator notes and pages from participant guides.

In Chapter 3, we address the concepts of centralized and decentralized programs. These concepts are especially important for those of you working in larger organizations; however, regardless of the size of your organization, you should be addressing items at the organization and unit levels. We also take a peek at a unit's onboarding program and, specifically, the importance of the preceptor.

Chapter 4
Evaluating an Individual's Competency

This chapter may be the most important chapter in the book, because at the end of the day your onboarding and orientation program should ensure that each new nurse is working in a safe and competent manner. The first thing we address is whether time-based or competency-based programs are more effective. We believe that competency-based is best; however, we also are well aware of organizational challenges, such as budgeting, scheduling, etc.

The remainder of the chapter is devoted to competence—what it is, what it isn't, how to evaluate it, and what to do if you are not seeing it. We make some distinctions between competence and confidence that we know you will find useful. Additionally, we delineate among cognitive learning, psychomotor skills, and affective thoughts and behaviors and provide some tips on how to teach each and how to evaluate each.

Chapter 5
Working With Orientees

OK, maybe this is the most important chapter! In this chapter, we identify several different types of orientees:

- The new college graduate
- The experienced nurse
- The nurse who is progressing quickly
- The one who has made an error
- The one who doesn't get along with his/her preceptor
- The one who has a learning style that is different from his/her preceptor
- The one who struggles with interpersonal communication
- The one who wants to quit
- The one who likely will not complete onboarding successfully

Whew! This chapter provides specific examples of what an orientee may do or experience and provides practical tips for what a preceptor and/or nurse educator can do to help the orientee be successful.

Chapter 6
Evaluating an Orientation Program

Chapter 6 looks at different models of evaluation. You will note some overlap of the models, and that is intentional. The bottom line with evaluation is that (a) you must be able to show that the orientees are successful after completing the program, and (b) the principal stakeholders can see that the program is efficient and cost-effective.

We provide examples of evaluation at the organization and unit levels to help you as you navigate the evaluation process. A key point in evaluation is that you must begin thinking about it during the Analysis phase, as Analysis is where you determine what you want people to be able to do better and/or differently as a result of your program. We have also added a new section on mentoring in order to facilitate new employees' success beyond the formal learning environment of orientation.

Chapter 7
Temporary Employees and Students

New to this edition, Chapter 7 focuses on how educators and preceptors can facilitate successful learning experiences for travelers, float staff, and students. While many teaching strategies from other chapters apply to temporary employees and students, some of the regulatory, documentation, and organizational culture specifics are unique. This chapter provides tips and strategies focused on these nuances.

Chapter 8
Regulatory Considerations

We would be remiss if we didn't include information for you about accrediting bodies, federal regulations, etc. This chapter highlights the importance of working with your Human Resource professionals as well as key pieces of legislation that may impact you and your orientees. We also discuss the importance of documentation and talk about when, where, and how long to make it and keep it.

Chapter 9
Practical Tips for Staying Organized

Juggling orientees, paperwork, and schedules can be overwhelming. In our final chapter, we provide easy-to-implement ideas for keeping your electronic and paper files organized. We also discuss ways to use email and calendar software to keep the schedule from getting the best of you.

We have also provided an appendix that lists some of our favorite books, websites, literature, etc. regarding onboarding and orientation. We hope that you find the book helpful, enlightening, and perhaps even a bit humorous from time to time.

As you can see from what we plan on covering in each chapter, we aim to provide a well-rounded approach to creating and sustaining high-quality orientation and onboarding programs that meet the needs of the individual, organization, and the patients they serve. By providing you with a combination of practical advice and theoretically sound recommendations, we intend for you to have everything you need at your fingertips to ensure a successful orientation and onboarding program.

Whether you're new to leading orientation efforts or a seasoned nursing staff development specialist, we think you will find this book a great addition to your personal library. Once you've finished reading it, we hope you'll have new perspectives, found a greater insight, or at least gained a few nuggets of how to do some things better. Regardless of what you discover along the way, we hope you enjoy the journey through these pages as much as we enjoy sharing them with you!

CHAPTER 1

Important Considerations for Onboarding and Orientation

Introduction

Hiring someone takes time, money, and your energy! You spend time:

- Making sure the job description is up-to-date

- Reviewing résumés

- Conducting telephone interviews

- Deciding who to bring to your organization for interviews

- Interviewing and observing the candidate in your "natural habitat"

- Deciding which candidate is the best fit for your unit, your team, and your organization

Whew! That *is* a lot of time and energy. So, now that the new person is starting, do you leave his or her success to chance? Really?!?! As Dr. Phil would say, "How's that working for ya?"

You would not have picked up this book if you didn't realize that there's something missing in the way you bring new nurses to your organization. Studies suggest that organizations retain new employees longer and those employees are more successful when they have experienced orientation and onboarding. Within nursing, reports at the time of this writing show that as many as 23% of new graduate nurses quit within the first year (Kovner, Brewer, Fatehi, & Jun, 2014). According to a white paper written by David Freeman (2013):

- Up to 4% of new employees will quit after the first day.

- Most employees make up their minds within the first 6 months if they want to stay with the organization.

- 22% of new employee turnover occurs within the first 45 days.

- Hiring costs are now estimated to be three times the employee's annual salary.

- With a good onboarding process, 58% of your employees can still be with you 3 years later.

You may be wondering what the difference is between onboarding and orientation. Technically, *orientation* is an event—from a half-day "here is the cafeteria" to a multi-day workshop. On the other hand, *onboarding* is a process that really starts the day the candidate accepts the job offer. We will talk about both the event and the process throughout this book, and we will refer to both terms somewhat interchangeably. Both play important roles in ensuring that your new hire is successful and stays with your organization. Laurano (2013) notes that "only 37% of organizations have invested in strategic onboarding for longer than two years" (p. 5). That means that about two-thirds of organizations are doing little or nothing to help their new employees be successful and/or to welcome them to the organization.

Pause for a moment and consider your first day on the job...or even your first day as a new nurse. You may have to reach back quite a way to rediscover those thoughts and feelings (especially if they were so traumatic that you *tried* to forget them). We bet the emotions you experienced then aren't too different from what new employees in your organization are going to experience. Therefore, use your own memories to set the stage or context for the journey on which your new employees are about to embark. We want to help *you* help *them* in making this one of the greatest journeys they will ever take.

We do want to highlight what we think works well and how you can integrate it into your organization. Let's contrast two different onboarding experiences to bring some of the things that work well to light.

ONBOARD OR OVERBOARD?

To help illustrate the differences between a "good" and "bad" initial experience (or if you want a little reminder of what starting as a new nurse might feel like), check out the stories of Nate and Ron, who started as new graduate nurses in two very different environments. Nate had a positive experience that contributed to his professional success and was effectively onboarded. In contrast, Ron received a less than ideal introduction to his organization and was, shall we say, overboarded.

Nate started as a float pool nurse at a large urban hospital. While he was initially frustrated by a lengthy organizational orientation before starting to work with patients, he was well-equipped with in-depth knowledge of the organization's mission, vision, values, policies, procedures, and processes. Once he was able to begin working with patients, he not only had an assigned manager, educator, and preceptor, but he also was immediately matched with a mentor who checked in frequently on his progress. Being a float pool nurse, Nate did not spend more than 2–4 weeks on one unit, which could have easily led to the inability to develop meaningful relationships with his colleagues. However, the structured assignment of key personnel and frequently scheduled progress meetings ensured Nate felt connected and cared for. He was also invited to social events occurring offsite, which helped him learn more about the informal culture. Multiple education modules and classes, while a seemingly impossible task at first, occurred throughout his orientation experience, and by the 6-month mark, he was not only knowledgeable of appropriate practices but also began teaching newer nurses. Nate was successfully onboarded and quickly became a leader in the organization.

Ron started as an emergency department nurse in a small rural hospital. Due to a staffing crisis in the department, the manager did not allow new employees to attend formal organizational orientation. Instead, Ron had to watch videos of recorded orientation sessions

Continues

in his spare time to learn about the organization's mission, vision, and values. Initially, Ron was quite excited that he was able to care for patients on his first day at work. However, the excitement he experienced during the first few days quickly faded because he did not have a consistent preceptor or mentor to assess his progress. No one was able to provide Ron with feedback, and he discovered that practices varied widely between nurses. A lack of classes and education modules meant Ron had to spend time off the clock looking for information from his nursing school textbooks. After 3 weeks, Ron's manager did a "drive by" meeting where she asked Ron if he would be fine without a designated preceptor starting the next day. Not feeling comfortable enough to verbalize his uneasiness, he complied. Then, 6 weeks later, Ron was working large amounts of overtime, had no meaningful peer relationships, and unknowingly performed many procedures incorrectly. Unfortunately, one of these procedures resulted in the death of a patient, and Ron decided not to return to work. Ron was overboarded, and he moved out of state to find a new job.

Although the negative example might seem a little extreme, we do hope it illustrates the impact that even small negative experiences can have on a new employee. This book is devoted to helping you with every aspect of your orientation program and hopefully turning your overboarding nightmares into onboarding successes.

The ADDIE Model

So, how do we get started on this journey of creating great programs? Luckily for nurses, there's a systematic approach to instructional design that is almost identical to the nursing process (you remember Assess, Diagnose, Plan, Implement, and Evaluate, right?). In instructional design, this process is called the ADDIE model (Figure 1.1). ADDIE stands for Analyze, Design, Develop, Implement, and Evaluate (Branson et al., 1975). This is a process used by instructional designers and educators to develop programs that meet the needs of their respective organizations. For our purposes, it will be used to create and/or modify an onboarding and orientation program.

NOTE

If you are looking for more information about ADDIE, check out this website: http://nwlink.com/~donclark/history_isd/addie.html

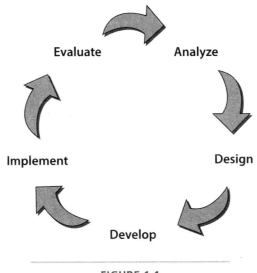

FIGURE 1.1

The ADDIE model for instructional design.

Analyze

In Analyze, it is important to ask the right questions. We will look at some key questions right now. In Chapter 2 we go deeper into this phase and discuss how to gather the data needed for an onboarding and orientation program. Once the questions are answered, it is time to begin the real analysis. Here are some questions to use as you finish data-gathering and begin to really absorb, sort, and make sense of the data.

- Who are the learners and what are their commonalities and differences?

- What behaviors and skills do you want to see them execute successfully?

- What constraints exist that may prevent them from performing successfully?

- What methods will you employ to help them learn and practice?

- What adult-learning theories might you need to apply throughout the program?

- What existing content and/or materials do you have?

- What is your timeline for completion?

Once you have the analysis done, you have a better understanding of the scope of the project. You have your parameters set and can start the next phase in the ADDIE model, Design.

Design

The Design phase is fun! When you think about Design, consider this story. Years ago, a new elementary school was built. School started before the fence could be built around the playground. Before the fence was built, the children stayed close to the school and the playground equipment. After the fence was built, the children played on every single inch of the playground. So, what's the moral of the story? Creativity needs parameters. You already discovered these parameters during the Analysis phase, so your creativity during Design must keep these parameters in mind. Some of them will include:

- **Learning objectives**—Does the program help the new employees meet the learning objectives of the program?

- **Scalability**—How easily can the program be delivered multiple times with small or large numbers of employees?

- **Pragmatism**—Does the program represent reality for the participants or are we taking them on a sci-fi adventure? Reality is best!

- **Cost**—How much does it cost per person. or per run of the program? Your leader will appreciate it if you can build a "champagne" program on a "beer" budget.

CHAMPAGNE PROGRAMS ON A BEER BUDGET

- *Reach out to other departments.* Often, the Staffing, PR, or Marketing departments will have "freebies" with your organization's logo imprinted. They may share those with you, and your new employees will love having some cool logo stuff!

- *Re-use content that already exists.* This saves you time and development dollars.

- *Small investments can save big dollars.* For example, buy a digital camcorder. Now, rather than paying for professional videos, you can shoot and use your own!

- *Go low-tech and get creative! You don't need a mannequin for practicing dressing changes when paper plates will work.*
- *Become friends with people in Central Supply! They often have items that are expiring that you wouldn't use on a patient, but your orientees could practice with those supplies.*

While many of you have looked at scalability, tend to be pragmatic (as most good nurses are), and are usually concerned about cost, we are guessing that writing learning objectives may not be something you do regularly or have done…ever. Learning objectives can be an art unto themselves. Here are three guidelines for developing good learning objectives:

1. **Action/task**—A well-written objective includes an action, that is, something that can be observed or heard. For example, "Administer medicine" would be part of a good objective because you can observe the nurse doing just that. "Understand policies" would not be a good objective because you cannot observe whether or not someone understands the policies.

2. **Performance measures**—What are the criteria on which success is based? In the example of "Administer medicine," we might add "within 30 minutes of receiving orders" and "at the correct dosage 100% of the time."

3. **Conditions**—Under what conditions will the action be performed? To complete our example, we might say, "Administer medicine at the correct dosage 100% of the time within 30 minutes of receiving orders during any assigned shift and unit."

CAN YOU FIND THE WELL-WRITTEN OBJECTIVES?

1. *Appreciate classical music by researching and discussing Beethoven's Fifth Symphony.*

2. *Update patient record within 30 minutes of seeing patient 100% of the time.*

3. *Communicate effectively with patient families 100% of the time.*

4. *Know how to deliver IV medication.*

OK, which ones are well-written? You probably guessed that the first one is bad. How can you measure someone's appreciation of classical music? You can't! Let's look at the other ones.

Continues

Number 2 is well-written. It contains an action "Update patient record..." a performance measure "...within 30 minutes of seeing patient..." and the conditions "...100% of the time."

Number 3 is well-written with the exception of the performance measure. How do we measure effective communication? We need more specificity on that in order to provide feedback.

The final one is bad. We cannot measure "know," we don't have criteria to determine success, and we don't specify conditions under which the action must be done.

The bottom line about learning objectives? They provide the roadmap for the Design, Development, Implementation, and Evaluation phases. If the participants don't meet the learning objectives, the program is unsuccessful...period.

WHAT DO THEY REALLY NEED VS. WHAT DO WE THINK THEY NEED

Robin and her colleague, Debra R. France, EdD, were asked to develop an orientation program for a company that had 30–35% annual turnover (by design). The company was a research and development consortium that brought together people from 14 different companies. These companies competed with each other in the marketplace but had to get along in the confines of the consortium. Robin and Debra had a challenging task.

Their analysis concluded that people needed to know what the culture and behavioral expectations were and needed an opportunity to practice them before being turned loose. They developed learning objectives that would meet these culture and behavioral expectations. Additionally, they found that much of the work was done in meetings. To this end, they developed a 3-day workshop called "Beyond Competitive Boundaries" that incorporated meeting skills, team skills, listening skills, and diversity appreciation. By the time they gathered all the content they wanted to use, they had about 10 days of content.

In order to make it work in a 3-day workshop, they got creative. They employed accelerated learning concepts to shorten the time needed to acquire skills. The design included putting participants into mock project teams (low-tech simulation); as the teams worked through the project, they were given opportunities to practice all the skills needed to be successful at the consortium. At the end of the 3 days, each team had to share with an executive what they had learned about the importance of collaboration in the consortium environment. Teams presented skits, taught the executives to line dance (it was the early

'90s), developed fun flowcharts, and came up with unique ways to share their experience. During the several years that Robin and Debra ran the workshop, they did not ever see the same presentation twice. Robin and Debra received the Corporate Excellence Award for creating the new and improved orientation program.

Additionally, there were 2 days that bookended the workshop. The first day had originally been a "death by PowerPoint" day that they changed significantly. They worked with the presenters (HR, Finance, IT, etc.) to develop creative ways of presenting their information (France & Jarvis, 1996):

- *To learn the building layout, they created a scavenger hunt.*

- *To learn the key HR policies, small groups were assigned different policies and had to teach each other about their respective policies.*

- *To learn about the harassment and discrimination policies, participants were given scenarios and asked to rate them on a scale. An employment law attorney facilitated the discussion.*

- *The last day of the week was devoted to safety training, as the consortium's site contained a clean room environment. The safety training was very hands-on, so it required little rework during the design process.*

Development

During Development, you start creating supporting materials and resources (paper and/or electronic), finalizing how different sections of the content will be delivered or facilitated, and finalizing the flow of the program. There are some basic things you need to consider during Development that will help you reach learners most effectively.

The first is the concept of flow. *Flow* means that you must arrange activities, lectures, demonstrations, etc., in a way that keeps the learners engaged and allows for the greatest efficacy. One way to think about it is from the perspectives of the facilitator/instructor and the student/learner (Figure 1.2).

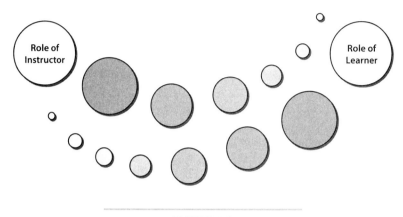

FIGURE 1.2

Role of instructor/role of learner in learning.

Debra R. France developed this model through informal conversations with students and facilitators of accelerated learning. At the beginning of a learning session, the role of the instructor or facilitator is large, as this is where the instructor explains and/or demonstrates what is to be learned. Note that as the process continues, the role of the student or learner becomes more prominent, so that by the end, the facilitator is providing feedback as the student demonstrates the new skill. This concept may be repeated over and over (micro-level) throughout an onboarding program and also at a meta-level as you design the entire program.

During Development, you will want to consider different methods for delivery of the content. These methods may include:

- **Instructor-led**—Used for group learning or one-on-one learning. Instructor-led modules may include lectures (less than 20 minutes in length), practice opportunities, etc.

- **E-learning**—This method is great for short bursts of information. Ideally, you would not want an e-learning module to be longer than approximately 45 minutes for organizational modules. Longer modules may make it difficult for the learner to stay engaged with the content. At the unit level, clinicians prefer shorter, 10-to-15-minute modules, as those are easier to work into their regular schedules. These shorter modules are sometimes referred to as *micro-learning*.

- **Job aids**—Provide step-by-step references for specific activities. Often, these are activities that are not completed by someone on a regular basis. An organizational example would be how to complete an expense report, which is something that most clinicians may not do on a regular basis. At the unit level, this could include how to dilute a rarely administered medication or how to document patient information in the electronic medical record. Most job aids are electronic and available via the organization's intranet.

- **Simulations**—Although many people think of simulations as high-tech, it is possible to have low-tech and effective simulations. In nursing, low-tech simulations may be as simple as practicing central venous catheter dressing changes using a paper plate.

Implementation and Evaluation

Implementation is where the rubber meets the road, so to speak. You have done your analysis, developed your learning objectives, and designed and developed a program to meet those objectives. You have created the appropriate materials needed. Now, all you need are your new nurses! For more on developing and implementing an onboarding program, see Chapter 3.

Evaluation is a critical component of the model and should be considered during Analysis and Design, especially. Evaluation should be conducted at the program level and the individual level. See Chapters 4 and 6 for more details about evaluation methods and models for individuals and programs, respectively.

ADDIE is a great model to use as you design your new (or improve your existing) orientation and onboarding program. It provides enough structure to keep you focused on your goal and allows for creativity in the design, development, and implementation of your program. You'll find that this book is laid out in a format similar to the ADDIE model.

Principles and Principals of Onboarding

With all these principles and principals about, you might feel like you're back in school. And, if you have never received formal training in managing orientation or onboarding programs, then to some degree, you are. In this section, we provide you with principles and principals of successful onboarding:

- *Principles* are the guidelines to keep in mind while analyzing, designing, developing, implementing, and evaluating an onboarding and orientation program.

- *Principals* are the key people who need to be involved in the development, implementation, and sustainability of the program.

Think of the principles as the foundation and framework of a building—if absent, the contents are exposed, unsupported, and likely to collapse. If we go with the same illustration, then the principals are the people who will inhabit, maintain, or provide resources for the building. All of these people will want (and need) to provide input into its construction.

We want to start with the principles of successful onboarding. Although we have divided these important components into two arenas, you will see overlap between the two—for example, engagement is part of implementation, but must be considered during design as well.

The key principles of onboarding are:

- Analysis and Design Principles

  - Answer the right questions with your process and program.

  - Be clear about job, team, and organizational responsibilities.

  - Leverage appropriate models.

- Development and Implementation Principles

  - Engage the employees each and every day.

  - Provide (and accept) feedback early and often.

- Evaluation Principles
    - Base the evaluation on the program objectives.
    - Evaluate the participants and the program regularly.

Analysis/Design Principle 1: Answer the Right Questions With Your Process and Program

Many orientation programs start with the premise that people need to know how to efficiently move throughout the building. Yes, they do; however, is that really the most important thing they need to know? Probably not. For your program and process to be successful, you need to start with determining the most essential prerequisites for a new employee, and that begins with asking and answering some very important questions.

For example, one question you might want to answer is, "What does it take for someone to be successful in this nursing environment?" This question will lead you to areas of regulations and compliance, as well as understanding the types of patients your organization assists and the organizational culture. To really answer these questions well, you will need to engage with the principals (key stakeholders). We will discuss different ways to engage with the principals later in this chapter.

We have provided several starting questions for you here (Worksheet 1.1), but feel free to modify these or add more of your own. As you are brainstorming which questions to include in your organization, if you find yourself debating whether or not to include a question, we would recommend you do include it here. Once you begin developing and implementing the program's components, it can be very difficult to return to the Design stage to make changes should additional information surface later. Asking more questions and gathering more information is best at this point in the game.

WORKSHEET 1.1 Key Analysis Questions for Onboarding

QUESTION	ANSWER
What does it take for someone to be successful in this nursing environment?	
How do we know if someone is successful within the first 30, 60, and 90* days?	
Whom do our new nurses need to meet within their first 30, 60, and 90 days?	
What additional skills or knowledge might they need within the first 30, 60, and 90 days?	
What do we already have in place to help them as they join our organization?	

Note: 30, 60, and 90 days are commonly used time frames in Human Resources for performance evaluations, but for training in highly specialized areas (such as an operating room or intensive care unit), longer time frames may be more appropriate.

We want you to look at these questions (from Worksheet 1.1) one by one to understand what type of information is requested.

What does it take for someone to be successful in this nursing environment? To answer this question, you will need a great deal of information about the work at an individual, team, and organizational level. A job description is often a good place to start. The challenge is to dig deeper with that question. Most of us have experienced working somewhere and feeling like we hadn't yet inherited the secret book of knowledge. That feeling has to do with the corporate culture. In *The Corporate Culture Survival Guide*, Edgar H. Schein (2009) notes that there are three levels of culture:

1. **Artifacts**—These are organizational structures and processes that you can see, but you may have a hard time understanding. For example, do people use titles, that is, "Doctor Smith," or do they use first names, and why?

2. **Espoused values**—These are the things the organization values and talks about. However, the actions of the people within the organization may not always support the espoused values. For example, to what degree should a new hire be able to align his/her personal work with the mission and vision of the organization?

3. **Shared tacit assumptions**—These are the things that are in that secret book of knowledge we just mentioned. For example, knowing that if Joe has shut his car door really firmly, you might want to avoid him for a couple of hours. Or, additionally, learning the financial and budgeting cycle so that you know when to ask to go to the next conference. Those are things that you may assume our new employees know, but they don't...yet.

Now that you've articulated the what, it's time to talk about how you know that someone is successful in this environment. How do you know? You know because the person is meeting and, likely, exceeding the job responsibilities (for additional information on assessing the ability to competently perform job responsibilities, check out Chapter 4 on assessing competency). You know because the nurse is interacting in culture-appropriate ways with patients and other staff. You know because Joe slammed the door, and your nurse waited until after lunch to approach him about the non-emergency situation.

Be explicit—very detailed—when answering the first two questions on the worksheet. If you can describe what and how the person needs to do the job effectively, you are well on your way to developing a great onboarding program.

The last three questions on the worksheet provide additional insight and information that you'll need to develop a great onboarding program:

- The first has to do with "who": whom your nurse needs to meet and when. It is easy to overwhelm a new person with (pardon the expression) "death by introductions." Really take the time to map out whom the new nurse needs to know and when. Start with the key staff in the unit and go from there. This could include fellow nurses, management/leadership, physicians, unlicensed assistive personnel, and ancillary staff (physical/occupational/speech therapists, respiratory therapists, child life specialists, chaplains, etc.).

- As you think about what additional skills and knowledge the nurse might need, keep pace in mind. The person is not going to be "perfect" on the job the first day...or even the 30th day, but you can start to identify the additional skills and knowledge the person will need: For example, in an organization where all staff are involved in shared governance, it might be important to have some knowledge and skill in meeting participation or even facilitation; however, the expectation would be such that someone new did not need these skills until after the 90-day onboarding period. Additionally, information regarding accrediting and regulatory bodies, such as The Joint Commission and the Centers for Medicare and Medicaid Services, and even including Magnet Recognition® from the American Nurses Credentialing Center, should be discussed, but again probably not until after the 90-day onboarding period.

- The final question might be one that many of you would want to pose first: What do we already have in place to support our new nurses? The advantage of asking this question last is that you are not boxed into the ways you have done things previously. By asking this first, you run head first into the wall of the existing orientation program and onboarding process. Answering this last allows you to answer the question from a different perspective, because the other questions have helped shape and change your expectations of your onboarding process.

These questions should be asked and answered by the principals—the key stakeholders in the process. We will have more on them later in this chapter.

Analysis/Design Principle 2: Be Clear About Job, Team, and Organizational Responsibilities

This should be easy to do, but it is not as straightforward as you might think. You started with a job description, which guided the hiring process. Most job descriptions include the ubiquitous "other duties as assigned." That leaves many questions unanswered for a new employee. Many larger facilities will have opportunities for nurses to serve beyond their daily job duties. Other duties may include serving on committees, collecting data for research projects, or serving as the chair for a fundraising campaign. Your new hires need to understand team and organizational responsibilities as well.

In Chapter 4, we reference a tool developed by Development Dimensions International (DDI) called a *Success Profile*. In that chapter, we use it to help you assess competency; however, if you have a Success Profile during the Analysis and Design phase, you can use it to help identify individual job expectations.

In addition to team and/or organizational goals (such as quality indicators or safety metrics), additional activities could include involvement in shared governance, improvement projects, and task forces, among others. If involvement in these groups is an expected behavior, that should be communicated clearly to the new employee along with *how* and *when* involvement begins.

Analysis/Design Principle 3: Leverage Appropriate Models

We have introduced you to the ADDIE model, and you will want to leverage other models to enhance your program. We have ones that we have found to be useful and we will spend more time on the models in Chapter 2, but we wanted to highlight that selecting the right models to use as you design and develop a program will be critical to its success. The ones we suggest are:

- Kolb's Experiential Learning Model
- Myers-Briggs Type Indicator (MBTI)
- DiSC/Extended DISC
- VARK
- AACN Synergy Model for Patient Care™

Develop/Implement Principle 1: Engage the Employees Each and Every Day

Employee engagement is a buzz-phrase that is probably a bit overused; however, given the statistics we shared with you earlier in this chapter, we believe that engagement is important each and every day. In fact, by working with your Human Resources and/or Talent Acquisition team, you can engage your new employees before they even start working. The time between acceptance of a new job and starting the new job can be a challenging time for your new employees. Reach out to them, and start talking about the onboarding process. Let them know how excited you are to have them on the team. Engage, engage, engage. You can do this by talking on the phone, inviting them to coffee, sending an email with their agenda for the first few days of work, etc.

So, what exactly does engagement have to do with onboarding and orientation? Well, have you ever participated in an orientation program and felt like you were sitting in front of talking heads who were just there to regurgitate information for your "benefit"? If you can make orientation engaging, you will be less likely to lose people the first day. Try to make even the basic stuff interactive and your new staff will love you and the job! For example, instead of simply lecturing through various policies and procedures, you could try using a case study approach where orientees break up into groups and are asked a series of guided questions that will require them to work through the policy and procedure manual. Or you can assign small groups certain key policies and procedures and have them "teach back" to the rest of the group. These are both more interactive methods to help new employees learn what can be a bit boring.

For the onboarding process, engagement should not really be an issue, but unfortunately, sometimes it is. In the book *How Full Is Your Bucket? Positive Strategies for Work and Life*, Tom Rath and Donald O. Clifton (2004) highlight the fact that disengagement costs U.S. businesses over $250 billion in lost productivity, illness, injuries, etc. And while it is not always about the money, most healthcare facilities want to have practices that will prevent them from losing money.

Did you know (Rath & Clifton, 2004):

- The number one reason people leave their job is because they do not feel appreciated?

- Studies suggest that bad bosses can increase the risk of stroke by one-third?

- 90% of people say that they are more productive when they are around people with positive attitudes?

Engaging people is not difficult. To help with this problem, you can try applying the golden rule, "Do unto others as you would have them do unto you," or the more profound platinum rule, "Do unto others as they would have you do unto them." In other words, treat people the way they want to be treated. This means that you find preceptors who are really interested in teaching clinical skills. You identify nurse educators who have a passion for learning, teaching, and helping others grow. These people will help keep your new nurses engaged. And, most importantly, you take the time to get to know each person as an individual.

We know that some of this seems very basic. However, employee surveys suggest that as leaders and educators, we sometimes fall down in the area of engagement. So, here are some simple things you can do to make sure that you are engaging your new nurses each and every day:

- Treat them with the respect they deserve, and they will reciprocate.

- Share the load—this person is not a nursing assistant. Do not ask them to do anything that you would not do.

- Answer questions in a respectful manner. Questions help people learn, and one of your most important roles is to help them learn.

- Make sure that you explain the "why" of a situation, if it is not self-evident. Humans are meaning-making beings, and understanding the "why" of any situation helps people put it in the right context.

- If you are someone who keeps a busy schedule, go ahead and begin blocking off time in your calendar where you plan to simply check in with the new employee, whether that's in-person or through an email or phone call.

Develop/Implement Principle 2: Provide (and Accept) Feedback Early and Often

Feedback is critical to success. It is critical to the success of your new nurses, and it is critical to the success of your onboarding program. That means that feedback is a two-way street. In order to facilitate that feedback, we want to introduce you to the EARS model. This model was co-developed by the co-author of this book, Robin L. Jarvis, and her colleague Debra R. France as a way for managers to provide employees with clear performance feedback. It has since been used as an interview methodology as well. The model (Table 1.1) can be used to give positive and constructive feedback.

TABLE 1.1 The EARS Model

MODEL	EXPLANATION	EXAMPLES
Example	A specific time or setting when the performance occurred (context)	*Positive or Constructive*—"When you were administering a medication to Patient X…"
Action	The specific behavior or action the person took	*Positive*—"you followed our medication protocol exactly." *Constructive*—"you did not double-check the medicine against the electronic medical record, per our protocol."
Results	The implications of the behavior or action	*Positive*—"This ensured that the patient got the correct medication in the correct dosage." *Constructive*—"Although you did give the right medication in the right dosage, you could have given the wrong medication."
Suggestions	An opportunity for you and the employee to discuss what worked well or what the employee could do differently next time	*Positive*—"You seem to have the protocol down, but I wanted to see if you have any questions about it." *Constructive*—"What can you do next time to ensure that you follow the protocol? How can I help?"

Providing this level of feedback helps the new employee understand what he/she is doing well and what specifically he/she can improve. We recommend sharing this model with your new employees and asking them to provide feedback to you in a similar manner. Their feedback can help you improve your orientation program and your onboarding process.

Evaluation Principle 1: Base the Evaluation on the Program Objectives

How will you know if your onboarding program is successful? You will have to evaluate it. On what do you base the evaluation? You developed program objectives based on the analysis you did, so using those objectives is the best way to evaluate the success of your program. You will need to determine how to get the evaluation information. You might use a combination of surveys, anecdotal information, and feedback from participants, preceptors, and hiring managers. There are several models for evaluation. We go into greater detail about program evaluation in Chapter 6.

Evaluation Principle 2: Evaluate the Participants and the Program Regularly

Because the purpose of the onboarding program is to prepare your nurses to work independently in their assigned unit, you will need ways to evaluate the participants as well. In Chapter 4, we look, in great detail, at ways to evaluate individual competency; however, for now, we want to talk about what it means to evaluate the program and the participants regularly.

In the Analyze phase, we asked the question about what success looks like for a nurse at 30, 60, and 90 days. The answer to that question provides a great basis for evaluating individuals throughout the onboarding process. The preceptor and hiring manager should be providing the participant with regular feedback about his/her progress and competency level. Chapter 4 is devoted to evaluating individual competency. Someone said that change is the only constant, and you should expect that with your onboarding program. At regular intervals—perhaps once or twice per year—you should evaluate the overall program. This will include what we discussed in Evaluation Principle 1, and we provide more suggestions for this in Chapter 6.

Principals

Principals are the people who are stakeholders in the orientation program and the onboarding process. They may include:

- Hiring manager
- Nurse educator
- Preceptor

- Unit nursing director
- Hospital/organizational nursing director
- Other healthcare providers
- Patient(s) and family
- New employee

Each principal will bring unique insights, experiences, and ideas to the party. Getting input from all of them will help ensure that you understand their expectations for the onboarding process. Obviously, this list was made from the perspective of a good-sized hospital. You will need to adjust your list of principals based on the requirements and structure of your organization. There will be different ways of engaging the stakeholders to get their input as well.

The hiring manager, the nurse educator, and the preceptor probably have the biggest stakes in ensuring the success of the new employee. The good news is that you probably have gathered their input if you applied Analysis/Design Principle 1 (answering the right questions) successfully. The questions from Principle 1 cannot be answered in a vacuum, so if you sought input, it was likely from these three people.

Specific information you can glean from the hiring manager should hit all of the principles highlighted earlier. The hiring manager should be able to articulate job expectations and responsibilities, how success is measured, and how frequently feedback will be provided. You may also bring in peers and other healthcare providers (such as physicians or ancillary staff) at this point to discuss what level of competence is required to independently and safely care for patients.

The nurse educator and preceptor are two sides of the same coin. Ideally, the preceptor is providing coaching and feedback on clinical skills in real time, and the nurse educator is facilitating sessions to help the new nurse be a better leader by focusing on some of the socio-emotional skills required to be successful. Although the educator may be found teaching clinical skills, this will likely be done in a simulated or classroom session.

Unit and organizational directors can provide "high-level" insight into how the mission and vision of the organization influence the expectations of an orientation program. Because organizations are constantly changing, these principals need to assess the current state of—and determine the future direction for—an orientation program as it relates to the organization's goals.

Conclusion

Remember, you have invested a lot of time and money to bring new nurses into your organization. Developing a great onboarding and orientation program will help ensure that your investment pays off. By applying the concepts presented in this chapter, you are well on your way to having an onboarding approach that is engaging and rewarding and one that will keep your new nurses excited about their roles in your organization.

Questions for Reflection/Discussion

1. Who are your principals for this onboarding program?

2. What are your next steps in working on the onboarding program?

3. If time and resources were not an issue, what would your ideal nursing orientation and onboarding program look like?

KEY TAKEAWAYS

- *Onboard, don't overboard, your new nurses!*
- *Apply the ADDIE model principles to make your process and program a success.*
- *Engage the principals early and often.*

References

Branson, R. K., Rayner, G. T., Cox, J. L., Furman, J. P., King, F. J., & Hannum, W. H. (1975). *Interservice procedures for instructional systems development.* (5 vols.) (TRADOC Pam 350-30 NAVEDTRA 106A). Ft. Monroe, VA: U.S. Army Training and Doctrine Command, August 1975 (NTIS No. ADA 019 486 through ADA 019 490).

France, D., & Jarvis, L. (1996). Quick starts for new employees. *Training & development, 50*(10), 47–50.

Freeman, D. (2013). *Onboarding and socialization for better retention.* Emeryville, CA: Cytiva, Inc.

Kovner, C. T., Brewer, C. S., Fatehi, F., & Jun, J. (2014). What does nurse turnover rate mean and what is the rate? *Policy, Politics, & Nursing Practice, 15*(3–4, 64–71). doi: 10.1177/1527154414547953

Laurano, M. (2013). *Onboarding 2013: A new look at new hires.* Aberdeen Group. Retrieved from http://deliberatepractice.com.au/wp-content/uploads/2013/04/Onboarding-2013.pdf

Rath, T., & Clifton, D. O. (2004). *How full is your bucket? Positive strategies for work and life.* New York, NY: Gallup Press.

Schein, E. (2009). *The corporate culture survival guide.* San Francisco, CA: Jossey-Bass.

CHAPTER 2

Analysis and Design of an Onboarding Program

Introduction

Now that you have some basic understanding of the approach and the key principles and principals, it's time to take a deeper look at the Analysis and Design phases of the project that you started looking at in Chapter 1. To really analyze what you've got in a program and what you want, and to position yourself to design a successful program, you need to:

- Collect data from the principals

- Assess any existing programs

- Understand your learners

- Consider how culture and connection will fit into your program structure

Only when you have taken these steps are you ready to make recommendations and move to design.

Gathering Data From the Principals

You'll remember from Chapter 1 that principals are the key people who need to be involved in the development, implementation, and sustainability of the program. There are various ways to collect the information you need from them. However, you will want to adjust your data-gathering method based on the principal involved. Table 2.1 highlights some data-gathering techniques and with whom you might wish to use them.

TABLE 2.1 Data-Gathering Methods

METHOD	EXPLANATION	PRINCIPALS
One-on-One Interviews	This method provides the greatest amount of anecdotal information; however, it can be very time-consuming.	Unit/organizational directors
Focus Groups	This method can be a great way to gather a lot of information. We recommend that if you use focus groups, you separate them by stakeholder group. Your groups should have at least five people and no more than nine or ten.	Hiring managers, preceptors, nurse educators, other healthcare providers, new employees
Surveys	Surveys can be used effectively if you have a large number of people and little time. They can be used to collect information from a more disparate group of individuals.	Patients and families, new employees

Interview Questions

When interviewing unit or organizational directors, you'll want to be sure to cover certain key areas by asking the following:

- What does success look like for a nurse on your unit?
- What are the most important behaviors you want to see from a nurse on your unit?
- What are the most important things (projects, success factors, etc.) that a new nurse on your unit needs to know?
- Who do they need to know?

You'll want to tailor other questions to your specific situation, but the questions listed above represent ground you'll definitely want to cover.

So, You Want to Run a Focus Group...

If you plan on using a focus group, Table 2.2 provides a suggested agenda as well as some facilitation ideas that you can apply. We recommend that your focus group have no more than eight to ten participants, and you should allow 90 minutes for the meeting. This agenda would work well with hiring managers, nurse educators, and preceptors.

TABLE 2.2 Focus Group Agenda

METHOD	WHO	HOW	TIME/TOTAL
Welcome	Facilitator	Discuss purpose Review agenda Review ground rules Introductions (if needed)	15 minutes/ 15 minutes
What does success look like?	All	Groups of 3 —Discuss —Capture ideas on flipcharts Large group —Group reports —Discuss —Agree	30 minutes/ 45 minutes
Who do they need to know?	All	Thought Gallery —1 flipchart each for 30, 60 and 90 days —Each participant gets sticky notes —One idea per sticky —Placed on appropriate flipchart —Discuss —Agree	30 minutes/ 75 minutes
What else do they need to know?	All	Discuss (capture on flipchart)	10 minutes/ 85 minutes
Next steps	Facilitator	Share with group Thank them for their participation	5 minutes/ 90 minutes

Conducting Surveys

You'll use surveys most often to gather information from patients and families and from new employees. Before we talk about survey questions, we want to talk about survey tools you can use, and what you need to know about writing surveys in general.

Most people are connected to the Internet, so we would recommend using an electronic survey tool. Many of these are inexpensive, or possibly even free, depending upon how often you want to survey, how many people you want to survey, and how much analytical support you will need. Some possible tools include:

- SurveyMonkey—https://www.surveymonkey.com/
- SoGoSurvey—http://www.sogosurvey.com/
- SurveyPlanet—http://surveyplanet.com/
- REDCap—http://www.project-redcap.org/

Once you have selected a tool to use and are ready to start writing the survey, here are a few suggestions that can make your survey easy to read, easy to complete, and useful for you:

- Have you heard of KISS—Keep It Simple, Silly? Surveys are no exception to this adage. Ideally, keep it to no more than two to three electronic pages, with no more than 10 to 12 questions per page. If it is longer than that (and three pages with 12 questions is getting pretty long), people will be less likely to complete it.

- Primarily count on scale-based questions, with a few open-ended questions at the end. If possible, use the same scale throughout the survey. Here are a couple of scales that seem to work:

  - 0 Not applicable—1 Disagree completely—2 Disagree—3 Neutral—4 Agree—5 Agree completely

  - 0 Not applicable—1 Dislike completely—2 Dislike—3 Neither Like nor Dislike—4 Like—5 Like completely

- Offer an out for the participant. Note that the scales above include a 0 for Not applicable. Give people the opportunity to not answer the question if it doesn't fit their experiences.

- When writing a scale-based question, make it a statement. For example, "The care I received from the nursing staff was consistent."

- Avoid questions that ask more than one thing at a time. You would not want to use, "The care I received from the nursing staff was consistent and they treated me with dignity and respect." These are two separate items.

- Use open-ended questions sparingly. Great questions to use include, "What did you like best about X?" or "What did you like least about X?" and "What would you do to make X better?" These allow the participant to provide meaningful feedback.

Finally, here are some questions you might want to ask a couple of groups impacted by the onboarding program—recent orientees and the patients and families they treated.

Sample questions for current and recent orientees:

- I received the training I needed to be successful on my unit.
- I met the people I needed to know to be successful in my job.
- I can articulate the expectations of this job.
- I know what the organization's mission is.
- I know what the organization's vision is.
- I can complete key procedures needed for patients on this unit.
- What did I need to know that I did not learn?
- What else would I have liked to know?
- I recommend that the following changes be considered…

Sample questions for patients and families:

- I was treated with dignity and respect.
- I received competent care from the nursing staff.
- I received consistent care from the nursing staff.
- I would recommend this facility to others.

Assessing Strengths and Weakness of Existing Program

If you have a program already, this section is for you. If not, you may wish to skip to the next section of the chapter.

Assessing the strengths and weaknesses of an existing program starts with Analysis, just like the ADDIE model shows us. Chapter 1 refers to key questions that must be asked as you design a program. You can ask those same questions and then compare your existing program to the answers. As a reminder, here are those questions:

- Who are the learners and what are their commonalities and differences?

- What behaviors and skills do you want to see them execute successfully?

- What constraints exist that may prevent them from performing successfully?

- What methods will you employ to help them learn and practice?

- What adult-learning theories might you need to apply throughout the program?

- What existing content and/or materials do you have?

- What is your timeline for completion?

The second thing you should do is look at the learning objectives of the program. Dr. John Sullivan, one of HR's "Top 10 Leading Thinkers," has developed 15 common errors to avoid in onboarding programs (Sullivan, 2008). One way to assess the strengths and weaknesses of your program is to use his common errors as filters. We have reduced the number of the errors he suggests by combining like errors. So, using Table 2.3 adapted from Dr. Sullivan's work, you can determine the strengths and potential weaknesses of your existing program.

TABLE 2.3 Common Errors to Avoid in Onboarding Programs

ERROR	BRIEF DESCRIPTION	POTENTIAL ACTIONS TO TAKE
Overloading new employees on day one	Providing too much information in a non-interactive manner	Use electronic tools for HR issues such as benefits enrollment, etc. Intersperse presentations with engaging videos of executives and other employees.
Being rigid about the time frame	Viewing onboarding as the first day or two at work—onboarding should last 6 to 12 months	Use a competency-based approach to ensure that each new nurse gets the right amount of tutelage and supervision.
Forgetting to take an integrated approach	Focusing only on organizational level, or unit level, rather than including team, individual, and/or department level	HR should provide the organizational level. Hiring manager, nurse educator, and/or preceptor provides the unit-, team-, and individual-level onboarding.
One-way communication	Asking for little or no input from the new nurse	Ensure that new nurse has opportunity to ask questions and provide feedback on the process.
No metrics or accountability	Providing no measures of success at any level of the program	Develop metrics that address things such as retention, hiring manager participation in onboarding, individual time to productivity, etc.
Ignoring diverse needs	Failing to acknowledge that your new nurses have different levels of experience, knowledge, and skills	Use a competency-based approach to ensure that each new nurse gets the right amount of tutelage and supervision.
Manager's expectations are unclear and presence is lacking	Not ensuring that the manager is present, communicates expectations, and stays in touch with the nurse educator, preceptor, and new nurse	Develop a checklist for hiring managers that provides check-in times/opportunities. Ensure that the nurse educator and preceptor communicate regularly with the hiring manager.

Continues

TABLE 2.3 Common Errors to Avoid in Onboarding Programs

ERROR	BRIEF DESCRIPTION	POTENTIAL ACTIONS TO TAKE
Lack of business case	Senior leaders (unit directors and above) do not understand the criticality of onboarding	Build a business case. Keep it current with quality metrics from your program. Get it in front of new leaders as soon as possible.
Failure to reinforce the organizational brand	New employees do not recognize the value that your organization provides in the community, and they can't articulate it to others	Ensure that the HR session includes corporate values, corporate responsibility platform, etc. If you have a Corporate Communications department, they can help make sure that your messages support the organization's brand. Have new hires practice a short (15 to 30 second) response to, "Why did you choose to work for X?"
Delays in offering onboarding	Asking new employees to wait until a certain number of new employees are available	Hold start dates until you have the right number of participants. This may be more relevant for new college graduate nurses than experienced nurses.

Adapted from Sullivan, 2008

So, now that you've gathered all these data from your principals and you've assessed what is and isn't working in your current program (if you have one), what do you do next? You take this information and analyze it so you can:

1. Come to some understanding about your learners

2. Consider what you need from your program from a 30,000-foot perspective

3. Develop some recommendations

The next sections dig into these next three important steps.

Understanding Your Learners

Before you dive into all the ins and outs of orientation and onboarding programs, you need to spend some time talking about the people who will be going through your program—your new nurses. And in the context of orientation and onboarding, you can more accurately look at them as your *learners*. We want to make sure that you keep your learners in mind during the entire process. To do that, you have to understand how they process information and translate that into learning. There are many learning-style models and theories out there, but we want to focus on just a handful that are easy to understand and translate into actions you can take as you build and implement your program:

- Kolb's Experiential Learning Model
- Myers-Briggs Type Indicator (MBTI)
- DiSC/Extended DISC
- VARK Information Processing Model

In addition to these learning models, we encourage the use of the AACN Synergy Model for Patient Care™ to consider the connection of nurse practice to patient and family outcomes as you design your program.

Kolb's Experiential Learning Model

The first learning style model we will discuss is David A. Kolb's model for experiential learning (McLeod, 2013). This model will provide a great foundation for you, as many of your new employees will (a) be accustomed to experiential learning, and (b) prefer it as a way to develop efficacy. Essentially, the model suggests four simple steps—that a person should:

1. Experience something
2. Be able to think about what he/she has experienced
3. Draw from that experience some knowledge or learning
4. Have an opportunity to apply the learning in a new and different way

Figure 2.1 illustrates Kolb's model, and the accompanying Table 2.4 explains the steps along with an example of administering an intravenous medication for the first time.

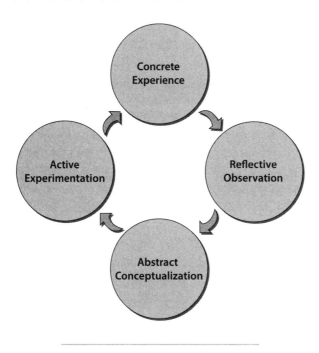

FIGURE 2.1

Kolb's Experiential Learning Model.

TABLE 2.4 Kolb's Experiential Learning Model

STEP	BRIEF DESCRIPTION	EXAMPLE
Concrete Experience	Doing or having an experience	A learner observes the preceptor administering an intravenous (IV) analgesic to a hospitalized patient experiencing pain.
Reflective Observation	Reflecting on and reviewing the experience	After observing the preceptor, the learner reflects on (thinks about) the event and the details involved.

TABLE 2.4 Kolb's Experiential Learning Model

STEP	BRIEF DESCRIPTION	EXAMPLE
Abstract Conceptualization	Drawing conclusions or learning from the experience	The learner begins to analyze and understand why the medication was given, why the IV route was chosen, how quickly the patient responded, how the preceptor organized the supplies, etc.
Active Experimentation	Trying out what has been learned	The next day, the learner attempts administration of an IV analgesic to a patient experiencing pain.

Keeping Kolb's model for experiential learning in front of you as you plan onboarding for your learners will mean paying attention to making the process experiential, while giving learners the opportunity to reflect and understand how they can take the learning and apply it in different settings.

Myers-Briggs Type Indicator (MBTI)

The second learning theory or model we will discuss is the Myers-Briggs Type Indicator (MBTI). Robin has been a qualified administrator and interpreter of the MBTI for over 15 years. This instrument was developed by the mother and daughter team of Katherine Cook Briggs and Isabel Briggs Myers and is based on the work of Carl Jung. There are four dichotomies in the MBTI, which allows for a possible combination of 16 types. Rather than chronicle the learning style specifics for all 16 types, we want to provide an overview of the dichotomies and address how these affect learning in Table 2.5. We are providing some definitions, as some of the words are not used in MBTI-speak as they are in regular conversation (The Myers & Briggs Foundation, 2013).

TABLE 2.5 Myers-Briggs Type Indicator

MAJOR AREAS	DICHOTOMIES	BRIEF DEFINITIONS	LEARNING EXAMPLES
Energy	Extrovert (E)	Draws energy from being with others. Talks to think.	Usually likes role playing and large-group activities.
	Introvert (I)	Draws energy from being alone or in small groups. Thinks, then speaks.	Usually needs time to think before speaking and prefers small-group activities.
Information Gathering	Sensing (S)	Gathers information through five senses. Likes details.	Likes processes and wants information in the correct order.
	Intuition (N)	Likes the big picture and takes information to form patterns.	Needs the big picture in order for the details to fit.
Decision Making	Thinking (T)	Makes decisions based on data and logic.	Prefers activities that include the data.
	Feeling (F)	Makes decisions based on values and impact on others.	Prefers activities that are people- or values-oriented.
Lifestyle	Judging (J)	Likes to make decisions and move to next item.	Likes activities that require decisive action.
	Perceiving (P)	Prefers to leave things open-ended in case more information is available.	Likes activities in which gathering data is more important than the decision.

The MBTI concepts are not only important when considering *your* presentation of material in a setting such as a classroom but also when selecting preceptors for your orientees. For example, if preceptors and orientees have fundamentally different approaches to decision-making (such as one being predominantly thinking while the other being predominantly feeling), the preceptor may perceive that the orientee is unable to make good decisions in the clinical setting. In reality, both approaches are valid (and some may be more appropriate in some situations than others, such as during end-of-life care), but there are fundamental differences between the teacher and learner.

DiSC/Extended DISC

A third model that helps people understand their own behaviors and preferences as well as those of others is the DISC. DISC is based on the theory of psychologist William Moulton Marston. Marston was a lawyer and psychologist who helped develop the polygraph test (he is also known for creating the character of Wonder Woman!). It is based on four basic traits—Dominance, Influence, Steadiness, and Compliance. Table 2.6 provides insights as to how to help orientees with the different DISC traits. Please note that all of us have all four traits, but one usually "rises to the top" as our go-to mode.

TABLE 2.6 The Four DISC Traits

TRAIT	DEFINITION	HOW TO HELP ORIENTEES WITH THIS TRAIT
Dominance	People with a preference for Dominance like: • To win • To get things done and quickly • To be in charge • To be right	• Orientees with a Dominance trait may want to begin doing things for themselves without you showing them. Discuss your teaching plan with them *before* jumping into it. • Let them do for themselves as soon as they are able. They will push you to complete orientation quickly. Use competency-based language to provide specific feedback about why they are not finished. • If it is an experienced nurse, you can refer back to your unit's or organization's policy and procedure manual to help him or her understand the consequences of not following policy and procedure.

Continues

TABLE 2.6 The Four DISC Traits

TRAIT	DEFINITION	HOW TO HELP ORIENTEES WITH THIS TRAIT
Influence	People with a preference for Influence like: • To talk through things • To influence others • To be active and lively • To have fun	• Ensure that this orientee has time to ask questions and engage in dialogue. • If time with patients is short, let the orientee know that he or she will get plenty of opportunity to get to know you and/or the patient and family better later. • Engage the orientee in meeting other new orientees and helping him/her build a network.
Steadiness	People with a preference for Steadiness like: • To focus on people • Harmony • To accommodate others whenever possible	• Ensure this orientee understands when and how to push back. • Help this orientee navigate the emotional "terrain" of your unit, as he or she worries about the feelings of others. • Allow the orientee to check with the patient and family about more than their basic needs.
Compliance	People with a preference for Compliance like: • To follow policies and procedures • To analyze data • To take a logical approach to just about everything	• Allow this orientee time to learn the policies and procedures. • Expect questions from the orientee when you do something that appears to be out of compliance. • Ensure that the orientee has the information needed to do his/her job.

There are several companies that sell DISC assessment tools and provide certification. They include:

- DiSC Profile—http://www.discprofile.com

- Everything DiSC—http://www.everythingdisc.com

- Extended DISC—http://www.extendeddisc.org

Robin has used various DISC profiles and tools. Extended DISC is what she currently uses. She finds their Work Pair Assessment helpful because it looks at two people's preferences side-by-side and identifies potential sweet spots for working together as well as potential challenges. Most DISC companies will provide team profiles in addition to individual profiles.

VARK Information Processing Model

Another model that plays well into the design and implementation of any program is VARK. Developed by Neil Fleming, VARK stands for Visual, Aural, Read/Write, and Kinesthetic (Penn State Learning Design Community Hub, 2010). It is a model that addresses how people process information most effectively and indicates how a person prefers to receive information. In Table 2.7, we provide insights into how to leverage VARK.

TABLE 2.7 VARK Information Processing Model

PREFERENCE	BRIEF DEFINITION	LEARNING EXAMPLES
Visual	Receives information by seeing it. Processes information quickly. Likes graphics.	Flipcharts and other visual aids help. Do not move visual aids to new locations (for visual learners, this is like shaking an Etch-a-Sketch).
Auditory	Receives information by hearing it—and being able to talk about it.	Tolerates "lectures" better than most; however, must be able to discuss what he/she has learned in order to cement the learning.
Reading-Writing	Processes information by reading it and writing about it.	May be willing to read aloud in class. Will want time to reflect and write in a learning journal.
Kinesthetic	Learns by doing and/or being emotionally attached to what is presented.	Let them "just do it!" When possible, help them feel the emotional connection of what they are doing.

A note about VARK—ideally, a well-developed program incorporates all four of these styles. Most people have a preference but can process information via the other methods as well. Only a few of your learners will require information be presented in their preferred way in order to comprehend the content. So, if you provide learning opportunities that incorporate all four preferences, your program should be successful and your learners should learn a great deal. For example, if you were teaching a class on the application of physical restraints for patients with psychiatric illnesses, you may want to present information in more ways than simply lecturing with a PowerPoint presentation (auditory and visual styles). You may consider incorporating time to practice the application of restraints (kinesthetic) as well as delivering a written case study requiring short-answer responses regarding the topic of ethical and legal considerations (reading-writing).

Of course, there are many other theories and models for how people learn; however, we believe that these four can have a significant positive impact in the development and implementation of the program and, most importantly, the self-efficacy of your learners.

AACN Synergy Model for Patient Care

Although it would be a great idea to include representation from patients and their families when making decisions about orientation design, it may be difficult to facilitate their presence at these meetings. Therefore, we propose using the American Association of Critical-Care Nurses (AACN) Synergy Model for Patient Care in consideration of the needs of patients and families, as it was designed to assist in demonstrating the connection between a nurse's practice and the patient's outcomes (AACN.org, 2017).

The AACN Synergy Model looks at matching patient/family needs and the characteristics and competencies of nurses. According to AACN.org (2017), "Synergy results when the needs and characteristics of a patient, clinical unit or system are matched with a nurse's competencies" (para 1). So, how does this affect the design of an onboarding program?

Based on the type of patients and care your unit is providing, you will need a certain level of competency. This should inform the length of onboarding and the type of additional training needed, as well as help you to identify critical success factors for your nurses. Check out Table 2.8 for more information on the various components of the Synergy Model.

TABLE 2.8
Definitions of the AACN Synergy Model Characteristics of Patients, Clinical Units, and Systems

CHARACTERISTIC	DESCRIPTION
Resiliency	The capacity to return to a restorative level of functioning using compensatory/coping mechanisms; the ability to bounce back quickly after an insult
Vulnerability	Susceptibility to actual or potential stressors that may adversely affect patient outcomes
Stability	The ability to maintain a steady-state equilibrium
Complexity	The intricate entanglement of two or more systems (e.g., body, family, therapies)
Resource Availability	Extent of resources (e.g., technical, fiscal, personal, psychological, and social) the patient/family/community bring to the situation
Participation in Care	Extent to which patient/family engages in aspects of care
Participation in Decision-Making	Extent to which patient/family engages in decision-making
Predictability	A characteristic that allows one to expect a certain course of events or course of illness

Source: AACN.org, 2017. Information in tables is retrieved from https://www.aacn.org/nursing-excellence/aacn-standards/synergy-model. Used with permission.

Table 2.9 provides definitions of the nurse competencies from the Synergy Model. These competencies were developed to illustrate how nurses can effectively meet the needs of patients. Therefore, these components could be the organizing framework by which hiring managers and unit directors set expectations of their onboarding program.

TABLE 2.9 Definitions of the AACN Synergy Model Nurse Competencies

CHARACTERISTIC	DESCRIPTION
Clinical Judgment	Clinical reasoning, which includes clinical decision-making, critical thinking, and a global grasp of the situation, coupled with nursing skills acquired through a process of integrating formal and informal experiential knowledge and evidence-based guidelines
Advocacy and Moral Agency	Working on another's behalf and representing the concerns of the patient/family and nursing staff; serving as a moral agent in identifying and helping to resolve ethical and clinical concerns within and outside the clinical setting
Caring Practices	Nursing activities that create a compassionate, supportive, and therapeutic environment for patients and staff, with the aim of promoting comfort and healing and preventing unnecessary suffering. Includes, but is not limited to, vigilance, engagement, and responsiveness of caregivers, including family and healthcare personnel
Collaboration	Working with others (e.g., patients, families, healthcare providers) in a way that promotes/encourages each person's contributions toward achieving optimal/realistic patient/family goals; involves intra- and interdisciplinary work with colleagues and community
Systems Thinking	Body of knowledge and tools that allow the nurse to manage whatever environmental and system resources exist for the patient/family and staff, within or across healthcare and non-healthcare systems
Response to Diversity	The sensitivity to recognize, appreciate, and incorporate differences into the provision of care; differences may include, but are not limited to, cultural differences, spiritual beliefs, gender, race, ethnicity, lifestyle, socioeconomic status, age, and values
Facilitation of Learning	The ability to facilitate learning for patients/families, nursing staff, other members of the healthcare team, and community; includes both formal and informal facilitation of learning
Clinical Inquiry (Innovator/ Evaluator)	The ongoing process of questioning and evaluating practice and providing informed practice; creating practice changes through research utilization and experiential learning

Source: AACN.org, 2017. Information in tables is retrieved from https://www.aacn.org/nursing-excellence/aacn-standards/synergy-model. Used with permission.

In addition, to bring the definitions of these competencies to life, the AACN also provides a few examples of what behaviors a nurse may exhibit depending on what degree of competency (using Patricia Benner's levels) the nurse has achieved. Benner's (1982) Novice to Expert theory outlines a continuum of increasing nurse competency that starts with Novice and Advanced Beginner. Nurses are rated on a scaled continuum of 1–5, but for purposes of this text, we have chosen to list only the first level, because it is the minimum level of competency that most would agree is needed to independently provide care. Table 2.10 provides these Level 1 characteristics.

TABLE 2.10
Level 1 Characteristics of the AACN Synergy Model Nurse Competencies

CHARACTERISTIC	DESCRIPTION
Clinical Judgment	Collects basic-level data; follows algorithms, decision trees, and protocols with all populations and is uncomfortable deviating from them; matches formal knowledge with clinical events to make decisions; questions the limits of one's ability to make clinical decisions and delegates the decision-making to other clinicians; includes extraneous detail
Advocacy and Moral Agency	Works on behalf of patient; self-assesses personal values; aware of ethical conflicts/issues that may surface in clinical setting; makes ethical/moral decisions based on rules; represents patient when patient cannot represent self; aware of patients' rights
Caring Practices	Focuses on the usual and customary needs of the patient; no anticipation of future needs; bases care on standards and protocols; maintains a safe physical environment; acknowledges death as a potential outcome
Collaboration	Willing to be taught, coached, and/or mentored; participates in team meetings and discussions regarding patient care and/or practice issues; open to various team members' contributions
Systems Thinking	Uses a limited array of strategies; limited outlook—sees the pieces or components; does not recognize negotiation as an alternative; sees patient and family within the isolated environment of the unit; sees self as key resource
Response to Diversity	Assesses cultural diversity; provides care based on own belief system; learns the culture of the healthcare environment

Continues

TABLE 2.10
Level 1 Characteristics of the AACN Synergy Model Nurse Competencies

CHARACTERISTIC	DESCRIPTION
Facilitation of Learning	Follows planned educational programs; sees patient/family education as a separate task from delivery of care; provides data without seeking to assess patient's readiness or understanding; has limited knowledge of the totality of the educational needs; focuses on a nurse's perspective; sees the patient as a passive recipient
Clinical Inquiry (Innovator/ Evaluator)	Follows standards and guidelines; implements clinical changes and research-based practices developed by others; recognizes the need for further learning to improve patient care; recognizes obvious changing patient situation (e.g., deterioration, crisis); needs and seeks help to identify patient problem

Source: AACN.org, 2017. Information in tables is retrieved from
https://www.aacn.org/nursing-excellence/aacn-standards/synergy-model. Used with permission.

It can be tempting to expect a new hire to perform at the same degree of competency as an experienced nurse in the organization, and the AACN Synergy Model can assist in designing a program that ensures basic competency without setting unrealistic expectations. While the discussion on assessing an individual's competency will come in Chapter 4, part of designing a successful orientation program is setting targets that are achievable, and the AACN Synergy Model may help you do just that.

Program Structure and the Four C's of Onboarding

Now that we have discussed the learner (the new employee) as the ultimate focus of our orientation and onboarding program, let's jump to a 30,000-foot perspective of orientation and onboarding. Talya N. Bauer, PhD (2012), has developed a model (Figure 2.2) for successful onboarding known as the Four C's. These are the building blocks for self-efficacy for your new employees.

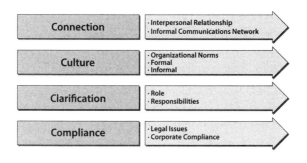

FIGURE 2.2
The Four C's of onboarding.
(Information in figure taken from Bauer, 2012. Used with permission.)

Keeping Dr. Bauer's model in mind as you consider design, development, and implementation elements will be critical in ensuring a strong orientation and onboarding program for your new nurses. Many programs do not include more than compliance and clarification; however, programs that include the culture and connection aspects will end up with more knowledgeable and engaged nursing staff. Including culture and connection should also improve retention of your new employees, because those levels provide more support on a personal and organizational level. The more that your new employees understand about the organization and what it stands for, the more likely they will be to work to support those values. Connection cannot be overrated either. In the book *Vital Friends* (2006), Tom Rath's research suggested that "while most companies spend their time thinking about how to increase an employee's loyalty to their organization, our results suggest they might want to find a different approach: *fostering the kind of loyalty that is built between one employee and another*. This is what keeps people in their jobs" (p. 58).

Making Recommendations

Now that you've reviewed the existing program, looked at your learners and their needs, and interviewed the key principals, you are ready to pull the information together and start making recommendations. If appropriate, you should make recommendations at the organizational and unit levels. Your recommendations should be presented to the key principals, with the exception of the new nurses, patients, and families.

You will develop a PowerPoint deck with your recommendations, if that makes sense in your organizational culture. If not, you might develop a short paper that highlights your key findings and the recommendations you are making. A suggested outline for the PowerPoint or the paper would be:

- **Methodology**—This should include your data-gathering process, as well as who participated.

- **Key Findings**—Based on the data gathered, what did you discover? This is an opportunity to introduce them to Dr. Bauer's model (Figure 2.2) and tie your findings to the four elements of the model.

- **Proposed Learning Objectives**—This will show the key principals what you plan to accomplish with the program and will make your recommendations easier to understand.

- **Recommendations**—Given the findings, how do you propose that the organization and/or unit should proceed? Again, you have an opportunity to tie your recommendations to Dr. Bauer's model. Don't forget to tie them to the learning objectives, too!

- **Call to Action/Next Steps**—What do you need from the key principals to proceed? Who will be involved, how much do you think it will cost, and how long will it take? These are the questions that your key principals will want to know.

Figures 2.3 and 2.4 show a couple of sample slides that might be in a recommendation slide deck.

Methodology

- Interviewed 10 hiring managers
- Interviewed 20 nurses new to unit within past 12 months
- Surveyed patients and families from past 12 months

FIGURE 2.3

Recommendation slide example 1.

Recommendations

- Develop 3–6 month onboarding process
- Include organizational level orientation
- Provide preceptor support
- Hire in cohorts to establish support network early
- Implement in Q2 next year

FIGURE 2.4

Recommendation slide example 2.

Designing the Program

Now that your recommendations have been approved, it's time to start working on the actual design of the onboarding program. You will want to review the big picture of your onboarding program and then start diving into each module, one at a time.

Over the years, we have used different worksheets to help us think through the design process. We have taken the best of those worksheets and put them together for you. As you begin the design, you will want to create design worksheets for each module. Also, you might create a meta-worksheet that highlights the overall goals of your onboarding program. When you have finished with design, you will have multiple worksheets. Worksheet Template 2.1 is a suggested worksheet for your use.

We wanted to provide you with a couple of examples as well. Sample Worksheet 2.1 looks at an organizational-level module on effective communication skills, and Sample Worksheet 2.2 addresses a unit-level module.

WORKSHEET TEMPLATE 2.1 Design Worksheet

Target Population Description	
Learning Objectives	
Delivery System(s) (Instructor-led, Simulations, etc.)	
Existing Content and/or Models and Theories to Use	
Materials Needed	

Sequence of Instruction (and Duration)	Topic	Method	Duration

Evaluation Method (should tie back to learning objectives and program goals)	Program: How will we measure the effectiveness of the program? Individual: How will we assess the new nurse as he/she moves through orientation?

SAMPLE WORKSHEET 2.1 Organization-Level Module

Target Population Description	New college-graduate nurses
Learning Objectives	By the end of this workshop, participants will be able to: Use an effective communications and delivery model to plan communications and select communication media; Present data and information effectively; Develop and deliver communications that positively influence others
Delivery System(s) (Instructor-led, Simulations, etc.)	Instructor-led with multiple practice opportunities
Existing Content and/or Models and Theories to Use	Joe Smith's presentation to AACN (May 2013) *Crucial Conversations* by Patterson, Grenny, McMillan, Switzler, & Roppe *Leading with Questions* by Marquardt
Materials Needed	PowerPoint deck with content loaded on laptop, Participant Guide, Evaluation Forms, Name Tents, Flipcharts with easel, Markers, LCD projector with screen

Sequence of Instruction (and Duration)	Topic	Method	Duration
	Welcome	Discuss Introductory activity	15 minutes
	Effective Communications	Mini-lecture Examples Your own case	30 minutes
	Influencing Effectively	Mini-lecture Examples Your own case	30 minutes
	Bringing It All Together	Prepare your case Practice with others Receive feedback	30 minutes
	Next Steps	Reflection Share	15 minutes

| Evaluation Method (should tie back to learning objectives and program goals) | Program: How will we measure the effectiveness of the program? Participants are 95% satisfied. (Level 1 evaluation) Their managers see improved communication and influence skills within 30 days. (Level 3 evaluation) Individual: How will we assess the new nurse as he/she moves through orientation? Participant is able to communicate and influence in a classroom setting using his/her own communication skills. (Level 2 evaluation) |

SAMPLE WORKSHEET 2.2 Unit-Level Module

Target Population Description	Experienced nurses new to a critical care environment
Learning Objectives	By the end of this workshop, participants will be able to: Identify "red flags" of impending shock; Describe common troubleshooting strategies for arterial pressure and central venous pressure (CVP) monitoring devices; Compare and contrast select inotropes and vasopressors
Delivery System(s) (Instructor-led, Simulations, etc.)	Electronic module and Skills lab
Existing Content and/or Models and Theories to Use	Unit-specific case studies *Essentials of Critical Care Orientation* (AACN)
Materials Needed	IV tubing & fluids, Pressure transducers, Patient monitor, Manikins, low-fidelity, Whiteboard & markers

Sequence of Instruction (and Duration)

Topic	Method	Duration
"Red Flags" of Shock	Online module	Pre-work
Introduction	Presentation of case study	15 minutes
Troubleshoot-ing Arterial & CVP devices	Didactic lecture Demonstration Hands-on practice	30 minutes
Inotropes & Vasopressors	Didactic lecture Low-fidelity simulation	30 minutes
Wrap-Up	Group discussion Paper evaluation	15 minutes

Evaluation Method (should tie back to learning objectives and program goals)	Program: How will we measure the effectiveness of the program? Participants are 95% satisfied. (Level 1 evaluation) Their preceptors see enhanced ability to manage patients with Arterial & CVP transducers as well as patients experiencing shock. (Level 3 evaluation) Individual: How will we assess the new nurse as he/she moves through orientation? Participant is able to demonstrate appropriate actions during the class's simulation & case study. (Level 2 evaluation)

Conclusion

If you take the time to analyze and design your program, the rest will come more easily. Take your learning objectives and turn them into design worksheets. This will make the development and implementation a little easier because you have the information you need for each module at your fingertips! You do not have to reinvent the wheel, discover fire, or develop a better light bulb! You have access to the AACN Synergy Model and other information that can guide what your orientation and onboarding program should be. In Chapter 3, we will help you take those design worksheets and begin to turn them into PowerPoint slides, facilitator notes, and Participant Guides. Let's go!

Questions for Reflection/Discussion

1. Who needs to approve the recommendations and provide the budget for this program?

2. What is the best way to present your findings and recommendations?

3. Who will help you with the design of the program?

KEY TAKEAWAYS

- *The old adage "garbage in, garbage out" is something to keep in mind while doing your analysis. Make sure that you have the right people engaged and are asking the right questions.*

- *You must understand how your learners learn in order to teach effectively. By using the models highlighted in this chapter, you should reach almost all your learners!*

- *Use the design worksheet—one for each module. This will help you stay organized as you get ready to develop the materials.*

References

AACN.org. (2017). AACN synergy model for patient care. Retrieved from https://www.aacn.org/nursing-excellence/aacn-standards/synergy-model

Bauer, T. N. (2012). *Onboarding new employees: Maximizing success* (SHRM Foundation Effective Practice Guidelines Series). Alexandria, VA: SHRM Foundation.

Benner, P. (1982). From novice to expert. *The American Journal of Nursing, 82*(3), 402–407.

McLeod, S. (2013). Kolb learning styles. Retrieved from http://www.simplypsychology.org/learning-kolb.html

The Myers & Briggs Foundation. (2013). MBTI basics. Retrieved from http://www.myersbriggs.org/my-mbti-personality-type/mbti-basics/

Penn State Learning Design Community Hub. (2010). Learning styles. Retrieved from http://ets.tlt.psu.edu/learningdesign/audience/learningstyles

Rath, T. (2006). *Vital friends: The people you can't afford to live without*. New York, NY: Gallup Press.

Sullivan, J. (2008, November 17). Onboarding program killers: 15 common errors to avoid. *ERE Media*. Retrieved from http://www.ere.net/2008/11/17/onboarding-program-killers-15-common-errors-to-avoid/

CHAPTER 3

Developing and Implementing an Orientation Program

Introduction

Some of you reading this book have the advantage of having an orientation and onboarding program already in place. Some of you do not, and that's why you picked up this book. Regardless of your situation, this chapter will help you develop and implement your orientation program. We will look at how to evaluate an existing program, explore organizational versus unit orientations, and then get into the anatomy of an orientation program for your new nurses.

Developing a Program

In Chapter 1, we introduced you to the ADDIE model. In Chapter 2, we walked you through how to analyze the onboarding situation as well as how to design a program by using worksheets for each module of the program you want to create. Now, you are going to use these worksheets to provide a roadmap for each particular learning module. Without this roadmap, you risk ending up at an undesired destination.

Once the module has been created, you must now develop any and all materials that you need to help your orientee learn. Using the examples we have provided here, let's talk about what you would do next.

The approach we have used in the past is as follows:

1. Review available content

2. Identify which content to use

3. Determine methods to present material and provide practice

4. Develop necessary supporting materials

The organizational-level module in this example is about effective communication skills. Let's pretend we have identified some existing content from a presentation that Nurse Joe gave at XYZ conference in May of last year, as well as two books we believe have good insights and tools for effective communication. We have decided which content to use and have contacted Joe to make sure he is OK with us using some of his PowerPoint slides.

As we determine methods to present the material and provide practice, we are drawn back to key elements from Chapter 2. We think through how to make it experiential, how to engage different thinking and information processing styles, and how to make it real for the participants.

We review the learning objectives to ensure that we are teaching them what the analysis indicated is important. By the end of this workshop, participants will be able to:

- Use an effective communications and delivery model to plan communications and select communication media

- Present data and information effectively

- Develop and deliver communications that positively influence others

We review our original thoughts about Sequence of Instruction (and Duration) and decide we are headed in the right direction. First, we have to get specific about how to carry out each method we have outlined. To illustrate, Table 3.1 expands on the example from Sample Worksheet 2.1 in Chapter 2.

TABLE 3.1
Detailed Action Steps for Organizational-Level Communication Course

TOPIC	METHOD	ACTIONS	DURATION
Welcome	Discuss	**Discuss** —Objectives —Ground Rules —Agenda	15 minutes
	Introductory Activity	**Introductory Activity** —Small Groups (3–5) —Answer: 　　Best communication experience 　　Worst communication experience —Large group debrief	
Effective Communication	Mini-Lecture	**Mini-Lecture** —Joe's slides 12–16 —*Crucial Conversations*, Ch. 2	30 minutes
	Examples	**Examples** —Working on policies committee —Draw some from class	
	Your own case	**Your Own Case** —Identify communication objective —Identify key barriers —Discuss with a partner —Large group debrief	
Influencing Effectively	Mini-Lecture	**Mini-Lecture** —*Crucial Conversations*, Ch. 7 —*Leading with Questions*, Chs. 4 & 5	30 minutes
	Examples	**Examples** —Working on policies committee —Draw some from class	
	Your own case	**Your Own Case** —Identify questions to use —Identify support you need —Discuss with a partner —Large group debrief	
Bringing It All Together	Prepare your case Practice with others	**Prepare Your Case** —Practice alone **Practice with Others** —Groups of three (3 rotations) —Large group debrief	30 minutes
Next Steps	Reflection	**Reflection** —Answer questions in Participant Guide	15 minutes
	Share	**Share** —Groups of three —Large group debrief —Thank participants	

Completing this detailed level of development is important for a few reasons. First, by including more detail, you can begin to see if the time allocations are correct. The more times you do this, the more comfortable you will become with time allocation. Second, you begin to identify specific tasks you want the participants to accomplish. Third, this level of detail will help you build the slides and facilitator notes as well as the Participant Guide.

Next, we have to build the supporting PowerPoint deck with facilitator notes, as well as a Participant Guide and any other supporting materials we might need. This becomes an issue of finding adequate time to sit down, start developing the materials, and get someone to help you review the materials. In organizations that are a little busier or that don't provide you with a quiet office, you may find working from a more secluded location may be beneficial in brainstorming and creating content for a presentation. If you are looking for secluded locations, we can recommend a nice corner table at your local coffee house. Also, you can schedule a meeting room at your facility, preferably far away from your regular work area. If it's a nice day, find a patio! Content development takes time and definitely is worth the effort.

Here are a few things to remember about developing content:

- Your PowerPoint slides should add to the experience, not detract from them. See the sidebar on PowerPointers for more tips.

- Write your facilitator/speaker notes as if someone who has never seen the content has been asked to facilitate. This will ensure that you get all the key points into your notes.

- The Participant Guide should not be a direct match to the slides. It should be a combination of what is on the slides and information in the facilitator notes.

POWERPOINTERS

We want to offer a couple of pointers about PowerPoint. Surely you have seen some not-so-great presentations, so if you want to create a more impressive presentation, you may consider the following tidbits:

- *People tend to put a lot of information on their slides. Remember that according to Cliff Atkinson, author of* Beyond Bullet Points *(2011), if everything you're going to say is on the slide, one of you is redundant!*

  - *A good slide should have no more than three to five key points, including sub-bullets.*

  - *In order to make sub-bullets worthwhile, you should have at least two sub-bullets. Otherwise, don't use them!*

- *We recommend that you do not go below 22-point font. Others might say 16-point, but we have found that keeping font size at 22-point or above helps keep you honest on the three to five key points suggestion.*

- *Never underestimate the power of a great photograph. For example, rather than putting the agenda on the slide, you could put a photograph of a map on the slide and talk about the agenda, then include the agenda in the Participant Guide.*

- *When selecting a color scheme, use complementary or contrasting colors (i.e., pick two colors on opposite sides of the color wheel).*

- *Avoid placing both red and green colors on the same slide because audience members who are color blind will be unable to differentiate between these.*

Figures 3.1 and 3.2 illustrate our take on what a slide with facilitator notes might look like as well as what the page might look like in the Participant Guide.

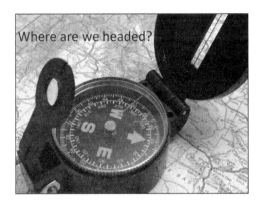

Say

Before we begin, I'd like to let you know where we are headed. If you'll turn to page 3 in your Participant Guide, you will find our learning objectives, agenda and ground rules for the day.

This module focuses on effective communication skills, including the ability to influence. You can see that you will get a chance to practice your own situation and we will discuss other examples as well.

Regarding our ground rules, let's agree that we will:
- Start and end on time.
- Respect differences.
- Participate fully.
- Turn electronic devices onto silent mode.
- Enjoy the process!

FIGURE 3.1

Sample organizational slide with speaker notes (displayed in Note view).

What you should notice about the slide and facilitator notes is:

- The photograph of the compass is a visual cue for direction.

- The title of the slide is consistent with the visual.

- The facilitator notes go into detail about the objectives, the agenda, and the ground rules.

Where are we headed?

Learning Objectives	By the end of this workshop, participants will be able to: • Use an effective communications and delivery model to plan communications and select communication media • Present data and information effectively • Develop and deliver communications that positively influence others

Agenda

Topic	Method	Duration
Welcome	• Discuss • Introductory Activity	15 minutes
Effective Communications	• Mini-Lecture • Examples • Your own case	30 minutes
Influencing Effectively	• Mini-Lecture • Examples • Your own case	30 minutes
Bringing It All Together	• Prepare your case • Practice with others • Receive feedback	30 minutes
Next Steps	• Reflection • Share	15 minutes

Ground Rules
- Start and end on time.
- Respect differences.
- Participate fully.
- Turn electronic devices onto silent mode.
- Enjoy the process!

Notes
_____
_____
_____
_____
_____
_____

FIGURE 3.2

Sample organizational Participant Guide page.

To help the participants, you should create a guide for them to use during the module. While the slide provides a visual cue of what is being discussed, the corresponding Participant Guide should provide the necessary detail. Notice that our Participant Guide example provides the detailed learning objectives, a high-level agenda, and the ground rules. Also, we left additional space for the participants to make any relevant notes.

Now that we have looked at an organizational-level example of a slide, notes, and the Participant Guide, we will look at a unit-level example (see Figures 3.3 and 3.4). Again, we developed this example specifically for this book. The unit-level example is about resuscitations for optimal results.

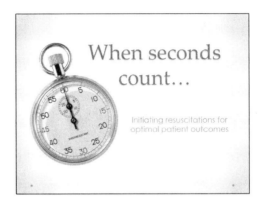

Say

Welcome, everyone! Today's topic will focus on the importance of timely recognition of cardiac arrests and initiating the emergency response system.

Go ahead and turn to the first page of your participant guide, and you'll find the learning objective, agenda, and ground rules. You'll see that we're going to spend some time discussing cardiac arrest situations, but the portion that most participants really enjoy is the end when we'll practice our new knowledge with a simulation.

Please review the ground rules, and let me know if you have any questions.

FIGURE 3.3
Sample unit slide with speaker notes (displayed in Note view).

The visual on this slide is perfect because the title of the module is "When seconds count…" The facilitator notes direct the participants to their Participant Guide for more specifics about the learning objectives, agenda, and ground rules. Does anyone see a pattern here? We do… what works for organization-level modules will work for unit-level modules. The concepts of the ADDIE model will work, regardless of what type of lesson you are designing!

When seconds count...

Learning Objectives	By the end of this class, participants will be able to: • Recognize signs and symptoms of impending cardiac arrest • Describe the nurse's role in initiating a resuscitation for a cardiac arrest • Identify unit resources for managing a patient in cardiac arrest before the code team arrives

Agenda

Topic	Method	Duration
Welcome	• Discuss • Share Previous Experiences • Introductory Activity	15 minutes
Resuscitation Procedures	• Lecture • Vignettes	45 minutes
Resuscitation Practice	• Code Blue Simulation	45 minutes
Next Steps	• Reflection • Share	15 minutes

Ground Rules	• Start and end on time. • Participate fully. • Turn electronic devices onto silent mode. • Enjoy the process!

Notes _____

_____

_____

_____

_____

_____

FIGURE 3.4

Sample unit Participant Guide page.

I DON'T WANT TO LECTURE YOU, BUT...

...some presentations can be dull and dry. Here are some ways you can keep your lecture component engaging and lively:

- *Your presentation shouldn't be just you speaking. Invite participation by asking questions or by having participants discuss something and report back to the larger group.*

- *Ask open-ended questions to get the discussion going. Use closed questions (yes/no) very sparingly, because they close down a discussion.*

- *If appropriate, include an activity; allow everyone to get up and move around at some point.*

- *Any "lecture" should be 20 minutes long or less. At that point, engage participants in an activity that is related to the content you just shared.*

- *Consider using videos where appropriate. When Alvin teaches other nurses about different types of seizures, he uses video to show the unique aspects of each type of seizure. A picture is still worth a thousand words!*

- *Use hands-on equipment if it makes sense. For example, would you teach someone about fire safety and not include a fire extinguisher?*

Programs With Centralized and Decentralized Aspects

The best onboarding program includes both centralized and decentralized aspects. That said, many of you may work for organizations in which you are responsible for the organization- and unit-level program, or you may be responsible for one or the other. Best practices would suggest that at an organizational level, you want to cover topics such as:

- Organizational mission, vision, and values

- Organizational culture—formal and informal

- Key HR guidelines and policies

- Facility tour

- Safety training

The benefits of covering these topics at an organizational level are tremendous. Your nurses will be meeting nurses from other units, as well as other key personnel. This helps build an organizational-level support system for them. Additionally, it's good to get interdisciplinary insights about the organization. In some organizations, this type of orientation will allow orientees to meet (or see via video) key executives.

At the unit level, you will want to cover things that are specific to your unit. These might include:

- Unit mission and vision (if available) along with outcomes data or performance measures

- Unit culture—formal and informal

- Unit-specific guidelines, policies, and procedures

- Unit tour

- Patient and family demographics

Most of you don't need us to point out the benefits of unit-level onboarding, but we will highlight a few for you. At the unit level, the culture might have a slightly different spin than at the organizational level, and it's important for your new nurses to understand these nuances. Also, your new nurses may never have worked with the types of patients you see on your floor, so this gives you an opportunity to help them understand those differences as well.

A huge part of onboarding is helping your orientees understand the organizational and unit cultures. As we all know, culture really has two elements—the formal and informal aspects. Culture is something that is difficult to teach; however, here are a few ideas:

- Formal aspects of the culture should be discussed early and often. These aspects include organizational- and unit-level mission and vision as well as organizational values and social responsibility commitments.

- Informal aspects of the culture might include items like whether you can call senior leaders by their names or their titles, and unit-specific things like the best way to approach your charge nurse and unit secretary when they're having challenging days. Are the doctors on a first-name basis with the nurses or do you call them "doctor"? What's the best way to let your peers know that you are taking a break?

- If you have people in a cohort, give them opportunities to meet and discuss what they have learned about the culture. These discussions probably will be focused on informal aspects of the culture.

- Preceptors should be prepared to answer questions about formal and informal culture in addition to questions about procedures, processes, and policies.

- Give orientees a chance in one-on-one situations to ask any question they wish. You can even provide suggestions of questions they might want answered in order to make them comfortable with asking these questions.

Nurse Residency Programs

Nurse residency programs (e.g., the University HealthSystem Consortium/American Association of Colleges of Nursing [UHC/AACN] Nurse Residency Program or the Versant Residency Programs) could be a great asset to you and your organization. These programs are primarily known for their ability to assist new graduate RNs in being successful during their first year in the workplace. However, these programs are being modified and expanded to include RNs who have moved to new specialties as well. By providing support and professional development activities for new employees, these programs appear to reduce turnover and increase satisfaction.

RESOURCES DESCRIBING THE BENEFITS AND DEVELOPMENT OF NURSE RESIDENCY PROGRAMS

If you're looking for a few references on the benefits of nurse residency programs or how other organizations have developed their programs, you might check out the following articles:

- *Letourneau, R. M., & Fater, K. H. (2015). Nurse residency programs: An integrative review of the literature.* Nursing Education Perspectives, 36*(2), 96–101.*

  This review article includes 10 outcomes-focused studies and 15 program development references. In general, new graduate nurse satisfaction and confidence increases with these programs, and retention rates are higher.

- *Kramer, M., Maguire, P., Schmalenberg, C., Halfer, D., Budin, W. C., Hall, D. S., ... Lemke, J. (2013). Components and strategies of nurse residency programs effective in new graduate socialization.* Western Journal of Nursing Research, 35*(5), 566–589.*

  This multi-site qualitative study identifies activities and procedures within residency programs that appear to increase their success.

- *Barnett, J. S., Minnick, A. F., & Norman, L. D. (2014). A description of U.S. post-graduation nurse residency programs.* Nursing Outlook, 62*(3), 174–184.*

  This multi-site survey study provides quantitative information on the characteristics of programs currently being used across many U.S. hospitals.

From a design and implementation perspective, a benefit of these programs is the amount of guidance provided to *you*, because a program structure is already outlined. These programs have a variety of curriculum pathways, evaluation surveys, course content, and evidence-based practice materials already created. For more information on these programs, check out their websites (https://www.vizientinc.com/Our-solutions/Clinical-Solutions/Vizient-AACN-Nurse-Residency-Program and https://www.versant.org/).

As an additional resource, we highly recommend Sigma Theta Tau's recent book *Developing a Residency in Post-Acute Care* (Cadmus, Salmond, Hassler, Bohnarczyk, & Black, 2017). The authors have written a very detailed approach to almost all aspects of a residency program. Even though they focused on the geriatric, post-acute care setting, the content can easily be applied to a variety of care settings. Check out Chapter 9 for a full reference to this book.

Anatomy of a Unit's Onboarding Program

By this point in the book, we've covered a lot of different principles, principals, methods, programs, considerations, etc. Hopefully, by now you have more of an idea of how to evaluate the onboarding program you currently have and design, develop, and implement the one that you need. This final portion of the development/implementation portion of the book is devoted to helping unit-based educators construct an effective onboarding program at the unit level. If you're more of a visual learner and want to see where we're heading, jump to the end and check out Figure 3.5 to see where these components fit into the orientee's overall experience.

Selecting Preceptors

Selecting a preceptor (or multiple preceptors) for a new employee can certainly be a bit stressful, because this decision will determine who his/her most significant teacher will be during the learning experience. There are many factors that influence selection of preceptors, and these could be simplified to include both the availability of preceptors as well as the professional development needs of nurses on the unit.

Availability issues could include:

- Lack of available preceptors if you are orienting a large number of orientees at one time

- Scheduling conflicts between orientee requests or classes and that of the preceptors

- Mismatch between the numbers of hours worked per week (for example, an orientee may be hired for full-time employment while the ideal preceptor works only part-time)

Professional development issues could include:

- Clinical advancement, because some organizations require precepting as a prerequisite

- The manager's request for the use of a particular preceptor based on recommendations from performance management

- Inexperience of a preceptor (e.g., some newer preceptors may be intimidated by having an orientee who has many years of experience in another area, or if a unit comprises primarily newer staff, it may be difficult to find a nurse with enough experience to serve as a preceptor)

There are also some situations in which both availability and professional development needs may play a role in the selection of a preceptor (some nurses who served as preceptors may become charge nurses and therefore unable to serve in this dual role). In addition to these, we're sure you could think of several additional problems in selecting ideal preceptors for your new staff. What follows are some key points we've identified that are important to consider when selecting preceptors.

From a practical perspective, you always want to select your preceptors as early as possible in the orientation/onboarding process. This allows you to *ask* the preceptors if they're able and willing to serve in this role rather than *telling* them due to last-minute planning.

TIP

Although each preceptor will have a different preference, we recommend asking the preceptor in person rather than through email or a phone call. Not everyone loves precepting, so although they may offer to do it, speaking with them in person allows you to assess any nonverbal cues that may assist you in providing the optimal amount of support for your preceptors.

Team vs. Individual Preceptors

Based on the unique combination of preceptor availability and professional development needs in your organization, you may be able to assign multiple (team) preceptors versus single (individual) preceptors to an orientee. There are pros and cons to both of these approaches, which we outline in Table 3.2.

TABLE 3.2 Comparison of Team and Individual Preceptor Structures

	TEAM		INDIVIDUAL	
	Pros	Cons	Pros	Cons
Scheduling	Allows the use of part-time preceptors	Requires availability of many preceptors	Easy to develop	May pose many conflicts with orientee requests and classes
Experience	Able to see multiple "ways of doing it"	Some items may fall through the cracks	Consistency in relationship (able to ensure progress)	Only exposed to one "way of doing it"
Preceptor Satisfaction	No single preceptor carries the full weight of teaching	Potential for conflict on team	Able to develop very strong relationship with orientee	No teaching breaks during orientation

Without knowing the unique situation in your organization, we recommend the team precepting approach. As long as you have enough preceptors to form teams, the benefits of this approach in overcoming the barriers of availability and professional development needs are substantial. Teams could comprise two to four preceptors (depending on hours worked per week, experience level, etc.), and ideally, the teams should remain exclusive and consistent (that is, preceptors are only on one team at a time, and they do not switch to another team with the next orientee).

Additionally, team precepting may actually enhance professional development of some preceptors because newer preceptors can be placed on a team with more experienced preceptors. This can decrease the stress of the newer preceptor (because they are not responsible for teaching the orientee everything they need to know) while providing a safe environment for receiving feedback (experienced preceptors can observe an orientee's performance and relay information to the newer preceptor).

Communication and Learning/Teaching Styles

Check out the potential preceptors' MBTI, DISC, or VARK results. Most people naturally teach in the same style they learn, so if you can match preceptors and orientees based on similarities, this may prove beneficial.

If the preceptor and orientee cannot be matched based on similar styles (due to a limited preceptor pool or a less-common style), you should anticipate that the preceptor might need more assistance or guidance with effective teaching strategies. Even experienced preceptors may encounter situations in which they are stumped regarding how to appropriately convey a concept. This could be due to a lack of training and development in effective and varied teaching strategies. Consider holding preceptor workshops for new *and* experienced preceptors to support their development.

PRECEPTOR WORKSHOPS

If you think your preceptors could benefit from some training and development of their own, you might want to hold a workshop or inservice for them. Here are some topics you could cover that preceptors are likely to find valuable:

- *Diverse learning styles (e.g., discuss the VARK theory and strategies for precepting an orientee whose preferred learning style is different from the preceptor's)*

- *Conflict management*

- *Giving and receiving feedback*

- *How to debrief an orientee following a traumatic event*

- *Evaluating competency*

For more resources on developing preceptors, you might check out Beth Ulrich's Mastering Precepting: A Nurse's Handbook for Success, *published by Sigma Theta Tau International (2011).*

Does the Preceptor Want to Precept?

We mentioned earlier the importance of *asking* preceptors if they're willing and able to precept rather than *telling* them they have to. But what if the preceptor responds with a big "No!" when you ask him/her?

First, explore *why* they are refusing to precept. Have they recently had a bad experience with an orientee? Are they serving as a primary nurse for a patient and don't want to take different patients? Are there personal reasons (for example, an ill family member or a divorce) that the preceptor worries will influence his/her ability to give precepting his/her full attention? Or do they simply hate precepting? Determining the cause of their refusal will help you find a solution, if possible.

Take for an example the preceptor who had a bad experience or the one who hates precepting. Perhaps his or her problems arise from inadequate development of his or her precepting skills? Consider placing them in a preceptor development course or working with them one-on-one to give them better strategies for working with orientees. You could also speak with his/her manager to see if this is a nurse who should not be precepting; if so, find ways for him/her to contribute to the unit through other leadership activities.

Similarly, if a preceptor has significant problems in his/her personal life, it is probably best to allow a break from precepting. If paired with an orientee, the preceptor may feel extremely dissatisfied with his/her work, which could influence the quality of learning the orientee receives. You should make sure the preceptor's manager is aware of his/her inability to serve in this role because this responsibility is likely in the employee's job description. However, it is important to be respectful of the preceptor's situation, and you can maintain a healthy relationship with the preceptor by discussing your desire to leverage his/her precepting capabilities once he/she feels well enough to do so again.

Finally, for the preceptor who is serving as a primary nurse, you must weigh the pros and cons of optimal preceptor selection and optimal nurse-patient relationships. This is likely a decision that needs to be made among leadership at the unit/department level, as it will influence both the quality of nurses completing orientation as well as the quality of care received by the individual patient who has a primary nurse. If a compromise could be made (e.g., the primary nurse serves as a preceptor but is able to be in close proximity to the selected patient almost every shift), that may be worth exploring.

PRECEPTOR POINTER: MANAGING YOUR ENERGY

What do you have the energy for? Being in a different season of life might mean you don't have the energy to invest in the primary preceptor role. Consider which level of teaching you could take on... If the primary precepting role is too much, try being a back-up or fill-in preceptor. You can still provide insight and guidance to staff while not taking on the responsibility of a new employee's entire orientation experience.

Regardless of why someone doesn't want to precept, if you are unable to change their attitude, we recommend not using them to precept, if possible. People who hate what they're doing probably aren't going to be good at it. The orientee may receive a better learning experience from a less experienced preceptor who loves doing it rather than a more experienced preceptor who is burned out.

PRECEPTOR POINTER: A CASE OF BURNOUT

Amy remembers her first new graduate nurse as being an extremely challenging teaching experience...

"The orientee was unable to acclimate to the complex and variable work environment of a pediatric critical care unit. I spent a lot of time providing emotional support, rather than serving as the teacher (which had been my precepting style with recent experienced nurses). After 12 long, emotionally exhausting weeks, the orientee completed orientation, but I was immediately assigned another new graduate orientee by the staff educator. The new orientee came to me terrified of this new environment, and because of the need to be tough with my first new graduate, I was insensitive to how truly strong her needs were. As a result, she came into our environment terrified and finished orientation terrified because I had so little time to reset my priorities between orientees.

"The second orientee was easy to teach and could have benefited from a preceptor to help her find joy in the critical care environment, if I had not made the mistake of jumping back in to precept too quickly.

"So I love teaching, but there have been seasons of my life where the energy it required to be fair to a new nurse in my facility was not something I had. Whether resulting from personal or professional reasons, I was neglecting my own professional development. If the educator had checked in with me each time she assigned me to a new orientee, it would have made me feel more a part of the process, rather than just being placed in an assignment because they felt like I could handle it. It ultimately wasn't fair to the new employee if I didn't have the required energy to give them all they needed to be successful."

RED FLAGS OF A BURNED-OUT PRECEPTOR

Watch for the following signs that your preceptors may be burned out or unfocused:

- *When asked if willing to precept, he/she hesitates or even provides nonverbal communication of disinterest (e.g., a sigh or an eye roll).*

- *When working with an orientee, the preceptor is found socializing or reading a book rather than observing and teaching the orientee.*

- *The preceptor frequently calls in sick or makes last-minute schedule changes on days when he/she is assigned to have an orientee.*

- *When the orientee performs a task incorrectly, the preceptor quickly resorts to verbal or physical abuse rather than constructive feedback.*

- *The preceptor is observed talking with colleagues about being "forced to precept" or "never being able to take care of patients by myself."*

- *Or very simply, the preceptor asks you for a break.*

Motivating Preceptors

On a more positive note, we want to discuss some ways you can motivate your nurses to serve as preceptors. It's not an easy task, so providing external motivators and facilitating internal motivators may help maintain a healthy work environment. Table 3.3 has some ideas to get you thinking.

TABLE 3.3 Preceptor Motivators

External Rewards	• Hold focus groups or send out surveys to determine desirable external rewards
	• Monetary incentives (e.g., differentials while precepting, bonuses upon orientee completion)
	• Organize appreciation events (e.g., schedule a dinner event off campus and invite key administrators to attend the event, too)
Internal Rewards	• Help preceptors realize the contribution they are making to the next generation of nurses (e.g., point out to them how the high-functioning nurses on the unit were previously orientees of theirs)
	• Provide preceptor development opportunities to make the experience more enjoyable
	• Encourage orientees to write thank you notes to preceptors upon completion of orientation

Introduction to Unit/Department

Once you've selected your preceptors, given your new employees their schedules, and ensured completion of central (organizational) orientation requirements, the orientees are ready to come to the unit! Before immediately placing them with their preceptors, you'll want to welcome them to the unit/department with an initial tour and overview. Just as the organization at-large has unique policies, procedures, guidelines, cultural nuances, and many new faces, so does the unit. If you place orientees with a preceptor and a patient assignment on the first day on the unit, orientees will lack fundamental knowledge to be successful (e.g., how to clock in, where to retrieve medications, and maybe even where to find a bathroom). Scheduling even a few hours to cover housekeeping and cultural issues will significantly enhance the orientee's experience.

Each unit will be unique in what should be covered, but here's what Alvin tells his new hires regarding what needs to be addressed: "The purpose of today's introduction to the unit is so that when you are with your preceptor tomorrow, you: (a) know where to go and how to get there, and (b) have everything you need to focus entirely on your patient assignment rather than worrying about getting lost or not having access to something important." You can see why the actual components could be unique to each unit. For an example agenda, check out Table 3.4.

TABLE 3.4 Example Agenda for an Introduction to the Unit/Department

Getting Around	Provide walking tour of unit/department, and be sure to include:
	• Break rooms and meeting rooms
	• Bathrooms
	• Lockers/showers
	• Manager, educators, and other administrative offices
	• Supply closets
	• Time clock
	• Where to receive assignment/report at beginning of shift
	• Fire extinguishers*
	• Gas shut-off valves*
	• Emergency exits & evacuation plan*
	Ensure access to secured locations and services (e.g., medication administration equipment, electronic documentation systems, supply closets, alternative entry/exit doors, etc.).

Continues

TABLE 3.4 Example Agenda for an Introduction to the Unit/Department

Socialization	Introduce new employee to the following people:
	• Manager
	• Educator
	• Preceptor
	• During walking tour, introduce to various other staff along the way
	• Administrative personnel (e.g., payroll specialist)
	Consider taking a photograph of new employee and having him/her write a brief bio to post for current staff.
Documentation	Complete, sign, and file:
	• Department orientation form* (typically, a checklist verifying discussion of policies/procedures along with various expectations of manager and employee)
	• Equipment agreements (e.g., pagers or keys), if loaning equipment from the unit
	• Unit-specific honesty, integrity, or HIPAA forms
Expectations	Discuss and/or set the following standards with the new employee:
	• Unit-specific policies, procedures, and/or guidelines
	• Unspoken or tacit rules (e.g., in which refrigerator should he/she place their lunchbox)
	• Requirements for completing orientation (target behaviors, learning activities, etc.)

*Those items noted with an asterisk may be a requirement of a regulatory body, depending on your particular organization. Refer to Chapter 8 or your specific regulatory body's requirements.

We recommend creating a checklist of the agenda you develop for your unit and keeping a signed copy of completion in the orientee's record. Doing that may help to demonstrate compliance with regulatory requirements.

TIP

Additionally, you may want to consider creating and maintaining a spreadsheet or checklist of your own that will ensure all necessary requirements and components of starting a new employee are covered. It can become overwhelming to verify receipt or completion of necessary paperwork, and keeping a spreadsheet will help you stay organized.

Time With Patients

Once an orientee has completed organizational orientation and received an introduction to the unit/department, he/she is finally ready to begin his/her precepted experiences and care for patients. Getting to this point may feel like an eternity for the new employee, especially if he/she is a new graduate nurse. This time (and especially the first day) is fairly exciting for most orientees, as it's the point where the rubber meets the road, so to speak. Although the preceptor and orientee begin to take the reins here, the educator and manager remain extremely important in this transition period.

We recommend checking in frequently during the orientee's first few days of taking care of patients to provide support to the orientee and preceptor, ensure the orientee has access to all necessary systems and equipment, and look for any red flags that may immediately surface. Whatever does surface, *do not wait* to address the situation. Even if the situation may work itself out, intervening early is always beneficial because it not only demonstrates support for the preceptor and orientee but also prevents wasting time if the situation needs escalation to more formal interventions.

THE TOP RED FLAGS
TO WATCH FOR IN THE FIRST FEW DAYS

During those first few days, be observant, and if you see any of the following red flags, consider quickly intervening:

- *Gross incompetence, carelessness, or negligence in the particular setting*

- *Orientee's verbalization of feeling he/she made a terrible decision to accept this job*

- *Atypical display of emotions such as crying or becoming completely silent*

- *Overconfidence displayed by the orientee frequently stating "I know that" or by attempting to perform procedures without supervision*

- *Calling in sick or not reporting in for an assigned shift*

- *Taking frequent breaks*

Educators and managers can help preceptors and charge nurses to select patient assignments that provide new learning opportunities while also reinforcing previously acquired knowledge. Due to the complexity of the healthcare environment and patient presentations, the learning trajectory is rarely linear. Preceptors may have to reinforce some concepts on more than one occasion. For concerns that arise, you may want to check out Chapter 5 for more detailed information on working with different types of orientees.

Other Learning Experiences

Although the majority of learning will occur while actually spending time with patients, other unit-based activities can be developed and implemented to augment patient care experiences. These could be taught by educators, expert or clinically advanced nurses, and even nurse practitioners or physicians. Certain limitations, typically financial, will always be present when augmenting patient care with these additional learning opportunities; however, well-designed activities are quite beneficial and a key component of most great orientation programs.

Classroom

Unit-specific didactic classes can be very useful for orientees, especially if they are conducted early in the orientation experience. We recommend providing only one or two classes per week because it is also important to have the opportunity to apply the information gained in class to the clinical setting. Beneficial topics for classroom content can be determined through speaking with key stakeholders, but general ideas include:

- Most commonly seen diagnoses or procedures

- Difficult, complex, or confusing skills performed on the unit

- Time-sensitive skills that should be explained before they are experienced in a clinical setting (e.g., resuscitation procedures)

- Situations that are emotionally challenging or difficult to discuss in the clinical environment

- Processes that preceptors may not have sufficient time to thoroughly discuss during a clinical shift

<u>**TIP**</u>

Consider partnering with other units to organize classes. This fosters interdepartmental relationships and offers orientees new insights or different perspectives on caring for patients. Additionally, it prevents reinventing the wheel if another department already has a well-designed class in place.

Skills Lab

Similar to the classroom setting, a skills lab provides orientees with the opportunity to learn and practice psychomotor skills without the fear of harming patients. You may want to include skills lab sessions as a part of classroom instruction (this helps to break up the didactic content and keep learners engaged). You don't need a physical room dedicated as a skills lab to provide excellent learning opportunities for new employees. You could find an empty patient room or bring supplies to a conference room or classroom. Orientees can benefit from things as simple as operating a peripheral intravenous catheter's safety device, drawing up unusual medications, preparing a drainage system for a chest tube, or even applying a 12-lead electrocardiogram to a female manikin.

Simulation

Simulation is becoming a big focus in healthcare education, both in academic and service settings. The opportunity to practice interdisciplinary teamwork, especially in rare or life-threatening situations, is a key benefit of simulation, and research is beginning to validate these benefits. Including simulation to practice skills such as resuscitation or end-of-life care can be invaluable for orientees.

Conclusion

This is probably a lot to take in, especially if you have no experience in developing an entire orientation program. While the previous content has focused specifically on developing individual chunks of an orientation/onboarding program, Figure 3.5 provides a generic timeline for moving an orientee from accepting a job offer to independent practice.

Before 1st Day

- Employee contacted by manager and educator (e.g., a phone call)
- Access requested for necessary systems & applications (e.g., electronic documentation, medication dispensing equipment, etc.)
- Necessary classes are scheduled, or the employee is registered for standing classes
- Orientation & onboarding schedule is sent to new employee

Organizational Orientation

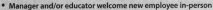
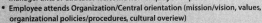

- Manager and/or educator welcome new employee in-person
- Employee attends Organization/Central orientation (mission/vision, values, organizational policies/procedures, cultural overiew)
- Employee registers for benefits & completes other HR forms (e.g., income tax forms)
- Tour facility & meet key executives
- Complete educational orientation actvities required of all employees (e.g., safety training, infection control)

Unit/Department Orientation

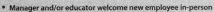
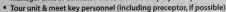

- Manager and/or educator welcome new employee in-person
- Tour unit & meet key personnel (including preceptor, if possible)
- Review of unit policies/procedures/guidelines
- Discuss expectations of unit/department onboarding

Unit/Department Onboarding

- New employee completes required education activities (classes, online modules, shadow experiences, etc.)
- New employee provides care for patients under preceptor supervision
- Regular meetings scheduled with the orientee, preceptor, educator, and manager

FIGURE 3.5

Timeline for orientation and onboarding progression of a new employee.

Questions for Reflection/Discussion

1. What challenges do you see in assembling and utilizing effective preceptors? What rewards could you easily facilitate for your preceptors?

2. What additional components should be added to the unit introduction for your own unit/department?

3. What role could you see classes, skills labs, and/or simulations playing in your orientation program?

KEY TAKEAWAYS

- *Set aside adequate time for developing educational content.*

- *Use the worksheet provided to help you develop specific modules for your program.*

- *Consider using a variety of teaching strategies that involve external resources, internal resources from other departments, and diverse educational media.*

- *Carefully select and adequately prepare preceptors for each new orientee because they will be the orientee's most significant teacher.*

- *From formal organizational culture to informal unit-based culture and everything in between, onboarding a new hire takes a large amount of planning and effort (but it's worth it).*

References

Atkinson, C. (2011). *Beyond bullet points* (3rd ed.). Redmond, WA: Microsoft Press.

Barnett, J. S., Minnick, A. F., & Norman, L. D. (2014). A description of U.S. post-graduation nurse residency programs. *Nursing Outlook, 62*(3), 174–184. doi: 10.1016/j.outlook.2013.12.008

Cadmus, E., Salmond, S., Hassler, L., Bohnarczyk, N., & Black, K. K. (2017). *Developing a residency in post-acute care.* Indianapolis, IN: Sigma Theta Tau International.

Kramer, M., Maguire, P., Schmalenberg, C., Halfer, D., Budin, W. C., Hall, D. S., … Lemke, J. (2013). Components and strategies of nurse residency programs effective in new graduate socialization. *Western Journal of Nursing Research*, *35*(5), 566–589. doi: 10.1177/0193945912459809

Letourneau, R. M., & Fater, K. H. (2015). Nurse residency programs: An integrative review of the literature. *Nursing Education Perspectives*, *36*(2), 96–101.

Ulrich, B. (2011). *Mastering precepting: A nurse's handbook for success.* Indianapolis, IN: Sigma Theta Tau International.

CHAPTER 4

Evaluating an Individual's Competency

Introduction

Having read this far in this book, you either already have a good idea of what it takes to build an orientation program, or you may already have an orientation program running (which may or may not be easily changed). Regardless, determining an individual's competency is the most pivotal moment during the orientation experience. This is the point where the new employee, preceptor, and other stakeholders decide if the individual is ready to practice independently. We identify this as the most pivotal moment due to the potential for harming patients if a nurse is identified as competent in his/her setting, when in fact, he/she may not be.

This chapter will explore various methods for assessing competency and the role of key stakeholders in the determination of competency. Your particular organization or unit/department will have to determine where to set the bar for what competency looks like, given your specific patient population. However, the tools for evaluating competency are universal; the goals you set or outcomes you hope to see upon evaluation will vary.

Time-Based vs. Competency-Based Programs

You need to determine whether you will use a time-based or a competency-based approach to orientation and onboarding. The camp to which you subscribe will be a fundamental decision in the design of your orientation program as it will influence stakeholder expectations, guide their actions, and help you to predict the allocation of an organization's resources.

- **Time-based programs** have a standard or pre-determined length of orientation, and those orientees who are not meeting desired behaviors are given a longer period of orientation.

- **Competency-based programs** have a length of orientation that varies based on the individual and the learning opportunities they receive.

Alvin's experience in learning how other organizations implement orientation is that most of them are time-based. Very few organizations have a competency-based orientation program in which orientation ends at the point in which desired behaviors are achieved. Figure 4.1 provides a visual representation of these two approaches.

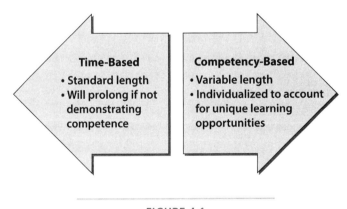

Time-Based
- Standard length
- Will prolong if not demonstrating competence

Competency-Based
- Variable length
- Individualized to account for unique learning opportunities

FIGURE 4.1

Approaches to orientation length.

We believe a competency-based approach is ideal because it allows for individualization of the orientation experience, which should result in more effective learning and, hypothetically, a more competent nurse. However, traditional time-based orientation programs may be difficult to change. Hopefully, we can convince you of the benefits of a competency-based approach.

What Is Competency?

Competency can be defined and described in a number of various ways, but we propose the following simple definition. *Competency* is the ability to perform the job tasks and duties for which one was hired. We believe this definition's simplicity allows it to be applied to multiple organizations and settings. This definition also means that when *you* are defining competency in your area, you will need to keep a copy of the job description on hand. Assessing competency can be approached through many mechanisms, and we have highlighted several of them in this chapter through exploration of the following considerations:

- Understanding competence vs. confidence

- Setting expectations before assessing competence

- Nurturing critical-thinking and interpersonal skills

- Recognizing the novice to expert continuum (Benner, 1982)

- Using learning domains (cognitive, psychomotor, and affective) to assess and teach

Understanding Competence vs. Confidence

As you evaluate your orientees, you must keep in mind the difference between competence and confidence. Although this may seem rather simple at first, distinguishing between the two becomes important in the event a new employee perceives his/her competence differently than the perception of others. For purposes of this discussion, we assume *competence* is the degree to which someone is able to practice nursing safely under various conditions, as measured by objective tools and/or other healthcare providers' observations. Conversely, *confidence* will be defined as the self-assessed (perceived) degree to which someone is able to practice nursing safely under various conditions.

We define these in this way due to the frequency with which these words are used among practicing clinicians and educators alike.

However, more accurate labels would be *subjective (self) competence* (instead of confidence) and *objective competence* (instead of competence). This labeling recognizes the value of the individual in assessing competence, an important activity for all stakeholders.

But we'll go back to using *competence* and *confidence* because these terms are more commonly used in the practice setting. Furthermore, for purposes of simplicity, we want to assume that both competence and confidence could be either high or low (knowing full well that a very large continuum could be constructed to indicate where someone falls on the actual scale). Using high and low as values, Table 4.1 highlights the four possible combinations of these two variables (competence and confidence) and what to expect in an orientee.

TABLE 4.1
Comparisons of Various Combinations of Competence and Confidence

		COMPETENCE (OBJECTIVE)	
		HIGH	LOW
CONFIDENCE (SUBJECTIVE)	HIGH	Both the individual and others agree that competence has been achieved. The orientee is ready to practice independently. **Action:** Complete orientation.	The orientee's perception of his/her performance is greater than that of others' perceptions. This could be problematic in the event an orientee is not receptive to feedback. **Action:** Provide open and honest feedback to orientee. Ensure all stakeholders understand expectations for demonstrating competency. Encourage reflection on performance.
	LOW	The orientee is practicing safely but doubts his/her own abilities. This could be problematic if the fear or anxiety is so great that errors occur due to this emotional distress. **Action:** Focus on growth, reaffirm strengths, and highlight performance so far.	Both the individual and others agree that competence has not been achieved. The orientee is either (a) still actively learning or (b) unfortunately working in an environment that may not be a good fit for his/her skill level and interests. **Action:** Continue orientation if actively learning. Consider transfer or termination if environment is not a good fit.

The ideal situations would occur when the degree of both confidence and competence are identical (both high or both low). Those situations represent expected positions in the learning trajectory. However, if the confidence and competence levels do not match, you might have some challenges. For example, if competence is high and confidence is low, patient safety is not of paramount concern but the employee's satisfaction with his/her job or role is. This may be a normal developmental phase for many new graduate nurses (for more information, check out the story of Moldable Molly in Chapter 5). The least desirable situation occurs when confidence is high but competence is low. An orientee experiencing this situation will require extra attention from preceptors and other stakeholders to become successful.

Competence and confidence—while both desired in practice and frequently interchanged in casual conversation—are two very different concepts. Being able to differentiate between the two, especially when there is a need for improvement, will be key in developing appropriate interventions to help the orientee.

Setting Expectations Before Assessing Competence

It is critical that the new orientee understand performance expectations from the very beginning of the orientation process. This helps you help them more effectively and efficiently. A tool we find useful in setting expectations is called a *Success Profile*. Robin's colleague, Jimmy Giles, has led global talent management and development for companies such as Fruit of the Loom and Goodyear. He adapted a tool that was developed by Development Dimensions International (DDI) by adding the key outcomes, goals, and deliverables of a job.

NOTE

In addition to the DDI, other companies that specialize in talent management such as Korn Ferry might have their own versions of a Success Profile.

What is a Success Profile? It is a one-page overview of key components of a particular position, such as a direct care nurse. A Success Profile identifies the ideal attributes that someone in this position would have. See Figure 4.2. It identifies the following:

- Key deliverables, or output of the job

- Knowledge and skills

- Experiences

- Competencies

- Personal attributes

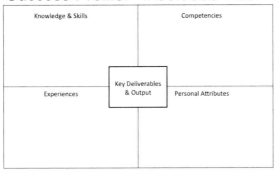

Success Profile: <Insert Job Title>

Knowledge & Skills	Competencies
Experiences	Key Deliverables & Output	Personal Attributes

FIGURE 4.2

Success Profile template.

How do you use a Success Profile in your organization? A Success Profile should be aligned with all the talent-management processes in your organization. A Success Profile can be used in hiring, setting performance expectations, individual development, and as part of the succession planning process.

For example, if you were to use a Success Profile in talent acquisition, you would have a recruiter screen for the left side of the profile—the Knowledge and Skills and Experiences you require. You would interview for the right side of the profile—the Competencies and Personal Attributes needed to be successful in the job. As Robin points out when she facilitates interviewing workshops, people are rarely fired for lacking the education or experience—they are hired for that—they get fired for "running with scissors" or "not being able to play well with others."

To create a Success Profile, follow the steps shown in Figure 4.3 and described in more detail in the next section.

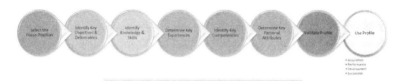

FIGURE 4.3

Steps to create a Success Profile.

1. **Select the focus position.** This is the critical first step! Identify the focus by a specific position, a function, or a level in the organization. Examples might include Charge Nurse (position), Nursing (function), or Executive (level).

2. **Identify the key objectives, deliverables, and/or outcomes for the position.** This does not need to be a laundry list of the tasks for a position, and it should not be a regurgitation of the bullets in the job description. This should be a high-level expectation of someone in this role. For example, if the position is for a direct care nurse, it might state, "Provides high quality care to patients and families. Participates in professional development activities that contribute to the organization's vision of continuously improving the quality of care delivered."

3. **Identify knowledge and skills.** Because a Success Profile is considered your "ideal person," list the educational requirements for the job, including those educational aspects that are preferred as well as the top skills that make a difference in successful versus unsuccessful people in that job. For example, a BSN might be required, but you would prefer an MSN.

4. **Determine key experiences.** Consider the Pareto Principle when thinking through key experiences: What are the top 20% of experiences that make 80% of the difference in being successful in this role? This might include experiences with certain types of patients, such as ICU, NICU, pediatric, geriatric, etc.

5. **Identify key competencies.** If your organization already has a competency model, then use those competencies. If not, your professional specialty may have suggested competencies that are critical to success. All competencies are important, but some are more important for a particular job. You want to identify the competencies that are most important for that job. For example,

a skilled nursing facility might place a greater emphasis on rehabilitation competencies, while a radiology department would place a greater emphasis on procedural knowledge.

6. **Determine key personal attributes.** These can be more difficult to identify, but you will know quickly if they are missing! Key personal attributes may include things like patient-focus or other intangibles that help ensure a person exemplifies what is important about your organization's culture. Some examples might include "focus on team's success over personal success" or "humble servant leader." Check out the upcoming section on "Nurturing Critical-Thinking and Interpersonal Skills" for some additional information on this portion of the profile.

7. **Validate the profile.** After you have created the Success Profile, you will need to validate it. Does it highlight the key aspects of the job description? Does it match expectations set forth in the performance review? Does it make sense to key stakeholders?

8. **Use it.** Finally, as mentioned before, the Success Profile can be used throughout your talent management processes. It only helps you if you use it!

Nurturing Critical-Thinking and Interpersonal Skills

An aspect of nursing that creates ambiguity in assessing competence is the need for orientees to possess and continue to develop critical-thinking and interpersonal skills. Like other healthcare fields, complex situations are almost a guarantee due to an ever-changing environment and nurse-client relationship. If nursing were limited to caring for value-free machines, the issue of assessing competence would be much simpler (which is actually the case when evaluating skills performed in a laboratory or simulated setting). However, the "real world" is much more complex and requires a balance of hands-on *critical-thinking and interpersonal skills.*

For example, inserting a urinary catheter into a manikin involves following a set of structured steps. However, inserting a urinary catheter into an irritable, febrile infant who presents to an outpatient clinic accompanied by four older siblings who want to "help" is a bit more difficult. It is this discrepancy between academia and practice that can make interventions and evaluation methods developed in the academic setting difficult to apply to the service setting.

Although we would love to provide you with a "magic wand" to help you teach and assess these critical-thinking and interpersonal skills, we only are able to emphasize that these are competencies that must be acquired before being able to practice safely. We don't have the space to define and describe these terms along with potential methods of evaluation, but there are critical-thinking measurement tools that exist (e.g., Health Sciences Reasoning Test [Insight Assessment, 2013]) and that can be created (e.g., situational judgment tests).

EXAMPLE QUESTION FROM A SITUATIONAL JUDGMENT TEST

You are currently caring for a six-patient assignment (maximum allowed per policy) on a busy surgical ward. One of your colleagues becomes sick and has to leave. You are told that you must take three of your colleague's patients. On a scale of 1–5, how appropriate are each of the following actions?

a.   Refusing to take report on the additional patients

b.   Calling the charge nurse or manager for assistance

c.   Delegating nursing tasks (such as medication administration) to the unlicensed assistive personnel

d.   Reprioritizing your tasks to accommodate the increased workload

e.   Asking the patient's family members to help with activities of daily living

f.   Delaying documentation in the patients' records until additional help arrives

Critical-thinking and interpersonal skills can be difficult to evaluate objectively because each nurse-client relationship will exist in differing situations. However, they are necessary skills, and we encourage you to delay an orientee's completion of orientation if you think his/her capacity for these skills is sub-standard. The important part is helping your orientee to develop in this area; here are some examples that may get you started:

- Administer case studies that focus on critical-thinking assessment (many books have been published to provide pre-made scenarios).

- Create simulated scenarios to evaluate and teach desired skills (these could involve as much or as little technology and simulators as you want).

- Focus on strengthening emotional intelligence.

- Converse with orientee and explore thought process through "What if…?" questions (e.g.. What if the patient had no breath sounds on the right…what would you have done then? What if the patient doesn't speak English? What if you were to get an unexpected admission? What if the catheter became clogged?).

CRITICAL-THINKING CASE STUDIES

There are many books available with pre-made critical-thinking case studies for various patient care environments. Some case studies are even available for free with a quick search in your favorite Internet search engine. Here is a brief list of books you might want to check out:

- *Melander, S. D. (2004).* Case studies in critical care nursing: A guide for application and review *(3rd ed.). Philadelphia, PA: Saunders.*

- *Harding, M., & Snyder, J. S. (2016).* Winningham's critical thinking cases in nursing: Medical-surgical, pediatric, maternity, and psychiatric *(6th ed.). St. Louis, MO: Mosby.*

- *Anker, G. M. (2011).* Delmar's case study series: Medical-surgical nursing *(2nd ed.). Clifton Park, NY: Delmar.*

- *Lunney, M. (2009).* Critical thinking to achieve positive health outcomes: Nursing case studies and analyses *(2nd ed.). Ames, IA: Wiley Blackwell.*

LEARNING MORE ABOUT EMOTIONAL INTELLIGENCE

Emotional intelligence (EI) comprises four pillars: Self-Awareness, Self-Management, Social Awareness, and Relationship Management (Goleman, 2006). Over the past few years, much focus has been placed on researching the connection between effective nursing practices and emotional intelligence. If you wish to learn more about EI, check first with your Human Resources department or Training and Development department. They might have coursework or reading materials available for you.

If you would like to learn more about EI in the context of nursing, here are a few relevant articles that may be of help:

- *Akerjordet, K., & Severinsson, E. (2007). Emotional intelligence: A review of the literature with a specific focus on empirical and epistemological perspectives.* Journal of Clinical Nursing, 16*(8)*, 1405–1416.

- *Aradilla-Herrero, A., Tomás-Sábado, J., & Gómez-Benito, J. (2014). Perceived emotional intelligence in nursing: Psychometric properties of the Trait Meta-Mood Scale.* Journal of Clinical Nursing, 23*(7–8)*, 955–966.

- *Freshwater, D., & Stickley, T. (2004). The heart of the art: Emotional intelligence in nurse education.* Nursing Inquiry, 11*(2)*, 91–98.

- *McQueen, A. C. H. (2004). Emotional intelligence in nursing work.* Journal of Advanced Nursing, 47*(1)*, 101–108.

- *Powell, K. R., Mabry, J. L., & Mixer, S. J. (2015). Emotional intelligence: A critical evaluation of the literature with implications for mental health nursing leadership.* Issues in Mental Health Nursing, 36*(5)*, 346–356.

For critical thinking, more specifically, it is probably quite a rare occurrence that an orientee has a significant problem with critical thinking if he/she were able to successfully complete his/her academic preparation and pass the licensure exam. Nevertheless, it is possible, so we have outlined an approach to evaluating and managing this possibility. This approach (the OPQRST process) is explained in Table 4.2.

TABLE 4.2
OPQRST Process for Approaching Struggles with Critical Thinking

	DESCRIPTION	RATIONALE
Objectivity	Explore objective accounts of concerning behaviors.	Presuming what the orientee is *thinking* before observing what he or she is *doing* could lead to inaccurate conclusions
Patterns	Look for a pattern or theme that occurs across multiple scenarios.	Assists with discovering the underlying problem while also considering the potential for situation-dependent factors
Qualify & Quantify	Qualify and/or quantify the impact these patterns could have on patient care.	Measuring impact will help you determine the severity of the problem but will also provide an answer to the "So what?" question if the orientee asks

Continues

TABLE 4.2
OPQRST Process for Approaching Struggles with Critical Thinking

	DESCRIPTION	RATIONALE
Reframe & Share	Help the orientee look at the situation from a different perspective (reframe) by sharing the emerging pattern or theme with the orientee.	Raises the orientee's awareness of the problem (althoughhe/she likely is aware of the problem) and helps explore why the orientee proceeded the way he/she did
Trial	Try alternative methods for approaching situations.	Helps the orientee discover that often there is more than one way to approach a situation, and can help him/her begin to make appropriate distinctions

Another excellent resource if you'd like to focus on improving nurses' critical-thinking skills is *The Critical Thinking Toolkit*, available from The Advisory Board Company at https://www.advisory.com/research/nursing-executive-center/studies/2009/the-critical-thinking-toolkit. This resource contains 16 activities focused on five different aspects of critical thinking. Activities include individual and group work covering topics such as detecting patient changes, decision-making, and communicating.

Recognizing the Novice to Expert Continuum

Patricia Benner's "From Novice to Expert" article, published in 1982, was monumental in describing nursing skill levels, and the model helps inform another aspect of competency—the idea that a new nurse cannot be expected to know *everything* at the beginning of his or her career. Benner's model outlines five major stages of skill acquisition: novice, advanced beginner, competent, proficient, and expert. You can read brief descriptions of these stages in Table 4.3.

TABLE 4.3 Patricia Benner's "From Novice to Expert" Model

STAGE	DESCRIPTION
Novice	• Non-experienced beginners • Rule-based, context-free decision-making
Advanced Beginner	• Marginally acceptable performance • Beginning to recognize patterns from experiences
Competent	• Actions are viewed in light of long-term plans • Well-organized and deliberate
Proficient	• Situations perceived as a "whole" • Decision-making becomes automatic
Expert	• Intuitively understands the entire situation • Has trouble articulating what is known due to the depth with which it is known

Source: Benner, 1982

Competence, as defined by Benner, is different from the definition of competency we are discussing in this chapter. Benner (1982) noted the stage of "Competent" was not achieved until one has been a nurse for 2 to 3 years (hopefully you won't have a new employee in orientation for that long!). For purposes of completing onboarding, you likely are looking for a nurse who has achieved the status of "Advanced Beginner." Keeping Benner's framework in mind will help you appreciate the development through which new nurses grow and may prevent you from setting expectations that are too high for new employees.

Using Domains of Learning to Assess and Teach

At this point in the book, we hope you have begun to appreciate the complexity of nursing orientation and onboarding as well as the varied approaches necessary to ensure individual competency. One simply structured method of performing this orientation and onboarding is to organize competency requirements into their respective domains of learning (cognitive, psychomotor, and affective). We label this as a simple structure because the learning domains lend themselves to evaluation using three simple questions:

- **Cognitive**—Has the orientee demonstrated he/she knows a sufficient amount to safely care for patients?

- **Psychomotor**—Has the orientee successfully performed skills that demonstrate the ability to safely care for patients?

- **Affective**—Are the orientee's words and actions congruent with the values and beliefs of both the organization and the patient population?

Cognitive Knowledge

Cognitive knowledge involves the ability to think, remember, reason, and problem-solve using one's mental capacities (e.g., recognizing a decompensating patient or calculating a medication dose). Measurement of cognitive-knowledge acquisition can be done through verbal or written methods but should answer the question: "Has the orientee demonstrated he/she knows a sufficient amount to care safely for patients?"

Cognitive teaching (and learning) can be facilitated through the following mechanisms:

- Instructor-led classes
- Online modules
- Assigned readings
- Observation of experienced nurses in the clinical setting

Cognitive learning can be measured through the following methods (among others):

- Tests and quizzes
- Question-and-answer discussion
- Documentation review
- Case studies

Psychomotor Skills

Psychomotor skills include the hands-on performance of tasks (e.g., obtaining vital signs or inserting a feeding tube). Measurement of psychomotor skills is done by observation of the skill. Assessment should answer the question: "Has the orientee successfully performed skills that demonstrate the ability to care safely for patients?"

Psychomotor skill teaching (and learning) can be facilitated through the following mechanisms:

- Observation of experienced nurses in the clinical setting
- Simulation scenarios or skills laboratories
- Online modules (especially if they contain pictures and/or videos)

You are a little more limited in the number of options available for measuring psychomotor skill acquisition:

- Direct observation of skill
- Achievement of desired outcome (e.g., verifying correct placement of feeding tube even though you did not observe the tube being placed)

Affective Thoughts and Behaviors

Affective knowledge is a person's integration of values, beliefs, and motivation. Facilitating, teaching, and evaluating in the affective domain is probably the most difficult of the three. Appropriate evaluation will answer the question: "Are the orientee's words and actions congruent with the values and beliefs of the organization, the employee, and the patient population?"

The affective domain is unique in that the methods for teaching also serve as the methods for evaluation. Some methods may include:

- Case studies
- Group discussion
- Guided reflection

EVALUATING AFFECTIVE THOUGHTS AND BEHAVIORS

Evaluating affective thoughts and behaviors is suited to the three methods of case studies, group discussions, and guided reflection. The nice thing about that is you can use the same example and apply it to all three methods.

Here is a scenario that you could use—a 3-week-old infant has been brought to the emergency department with a potential for having been abused by the mother's boyfriend. Both the mother and the boyfriend brought the baby into the ED and want to be present with the child. Hospital policy does not restrict visitation until an arrest has been made. You are the nurse caring for the child.

- *How would you handle this situation?*
- *What do you anticipate your conversation with the mother and boyfriend will be like?*
- *Will you treat them differently than other visitors?*
- *How should/would the care of the patient be different?*
- *What support systems have you identified for yourself to help you through this situation?*

As you can see, you could write this up as a case study for individuals to complete, use it for group discussion, or ask orientees to reflect on the case and write their answers to the questions.

Roles of Stakeholders (Principals)

Now that you have a better idea of what competency is and how it's measured, it's time to turn our focus onto what roles the stakeholders play in both measuring and facilitating an orientee's competency. These roles may overlap (especially as different organizations have different resources, job titles, etc.). We provide a generic description for each role, but you could easily shift these roles and responsibilities to other stakeholders.

Manager

Ultimately, the manager is the person responsible for competency assessment. Managers may delegate this responsibility to an educator or someone who observes the orientee more frequently (especially in organizations that have unit-based educators). However, from a regulatory perspective, the manager is responsible for the competency of all of his/her employees.

So, what are practical things a manager can do to assess an orientee's competency? Here are some possible activities:

- Check in with the orientee frequently and ask how he/she is feeling

- When seeing the orientee in the clinical setting, ask questions about the patient assignment to determine his/her understanding of the situation (e.g., "What's going on with your patient today?")

- Review, sign, and maintain orientation documentation upon completion of orientation

- Maintain regular communication with preceptor(s) and/or educator

It may be helpful to schedule meetings at regular intervals (e.g., every 2 weeks or every month) where the manager, educator, preceptor, and orientee can also sit down together to discuss the orientee's progress. Benefits of organizing a meeting in this way include:

- Providing a more formal feedback environment

- Ensuring all primary stakeholders are on the same page

- Demonstrating to the orientee that he/she is valued enough by the manager to block out dedicated time just for that individual

- Offering an opportunity for all stakeholders to review and sign relevant orientation paperwork

Educator

In organizations with unit-based educators, those educators will likely be the primary contact persons for most orientation-related activities, including the documentation and determination of competency achievement. (For information on documentation specifics, check out Chapter 8.) Therefore, the educator will be involved in a wide variety of activities that may assist with obtaining competency but should also be used to evaluate competency. For example, an educator may teach a class for new employees, and during this time, question-and-answer discussions or tests and quizzes could be used to ensure knowledge acquisition.

Not all organizations have a unit-based educator, and therefore, a manager or another designated staff member might perform these duties. Some units have a "lead preceptor" who oversees orientation activities, and the Clinical Nurse Leader (CNL) role is becoming increasingly popular. A CNL focuses on improving quality of care at the micro-system (i.e., unit) level. Although educating nurses is not a fundamental aspect of their practice (American Association of Colleges of Nursing, 2013), a CNL's leadership skills and advanced degree can make him/her an excellent candidate for conducting several of the orientee assessment activities that an educator might perform.

An educator (as well as the manager, lead preceptor, or CNL) may be involved in any of the following; however, this list is not exhaustive:

- Check in with the orientee and preceptor(s) frequently and ask how they are feeling

- When seeing the orientee in the clinical setting, ask questions about the patient assignment to determine his/her understanding of the situation (e.g., "What's going on with your patient today?")

- Review and sign orientation documentation from preceptor

- Aggregate all relevant documentation into one document for manager to review, sign, and file

- Maintain regular communication with preceptor(s) and manager

- Develop and deliver non-clinical learning opportunities (e.g., classes, simulations, debriefing sessions)

- Assign orientee to appropriate preceptor(s)

- If time permits, act as preceptor for one or more shifts

CHECK-IN QUESTIONS

Here are some questions that the manager and educator can use when checking with the orientee:

- *What's going on with your patient today?*

- *How's the family doing?*

- *What's keeping your patient here?*

- *What else do you have planned for the day?*

- *Are you getting the support you need to be successful with this patient?*

- *What can I do to help you?*

Preceptor

The preceptor will be the primary teacher/instructor during unit-level orientation. Because of this, the preceptor also serves as the primary evaluator of an orientee's competence. This is not an easy task; it requires skill, hard work, and compassion. Simply being an excellent clinician does not ensure you will be an excellent teacher, and many times, newer preceptors require a significant amount of professional development. Professional development specialists and managers will be essential in providing these development opportunities for preceptors.

The major responsibilities of the preceptor include:

- Collaborate with charge nurse to select patient assignments that will provide optimal learning opportunities

- Assess orientee performance on a day-to-day (or even minute-to-minute) basis

- Provide real-time feedback to orientee (both positive and constructive)

- Maintain regular communication with manager and educator

- Document relevant learning opportunities

- Review and sign final orientation document

Providing "optimal learning opportunities" can be challenging, especially in situations in which multiple orientees are on the unit at the same time or when selection of desired patients is not possible. *Mastering Precepting: A Nurse's Handbook for Success* (Ulrich, 2011) is another book published by Sigma Theta Tau International that provides much greater insight and detail than we can provide here. But in an effort to provide some practical information (and because you may not want to go online and purchase *Mastering Precepting* while you're in the middle of reading this chapter), here is a short worksheet that may help preceptors in choosing appropriate assignments.

WORKSHEET 4.1
Selecting Patient Assignments to Enhance Learning Opportunities

ORIENTEE NAME:

ASSESSMENT	CONSIDERATION FOR ASSIGNMENT
What are the orientee's primary strengths?	You probably want to avoid patient assignments that would be too easy for the orientee, because these do not provide new learning opportunities but rather reinforcement of previously acquired knowledge. (However, if an orientee is struggling with *confidence*, this could be appropriate to help enhance his or her self-esteem.)
What are the orientee's primary areas for improvement? (What has he/she struggled with or verbalized as being a problem?)	Selecting assignments that allow the orientee to work on areas for improvement with the assistance of his/her preceptor is ideal. Identifying these areas and transforming them into strengths is a key purpose of the orientation process. *Note:* Sometimes you can find an assignment that allows the orientee to demonstrate his/her strength while learning or improving another competency area. This helps the orientee with confidence yet continues to develop competence.
Has the orientee recently had non-clinical learning activities such as classes or workshops?	Selecting diagnoses and procedures similar to what was covered in the non-clinical activity would help to reinforce that content and helps many orientees to have those "ah-ha!" moments by providing the opportunity to see/touch/experience the information in real life.
Is there any patient with a rare diagnosis on the unit?	If less-commonly seen diagnoses or procedures are present on the unit, these could be beneficial to experience during orientation so that the first time an orientee provides care for this diagnosis or procedure is before he/she is working independently.

Documentation of relevant learning opportunities could include a wide variety of details, and Chapter 8 provides additional information. Briefly, however, a preceptor should document each shift:

- Assignment details (patient's age, diagnoses, procedures, etc.)
- Skills performed by the orientee
- Orientee's strengths and areas for improvement

Orientee

Unfortunately, it can be easy to forget the orientee's responsibility in assessing competency. The subjective experience of the orientee (as described in Table 4.1) is important in determining readiness to practice independently. Here are the activities in which the orientee should be actively participating:

- Verbalize expectations of preceptor(s), educator, and/or manager regarding what the orientee needs to feel successful
- Contribute to, review, and sign orientation documentation
- Attend and participant in all clinical and non-clinical learning opportunities
- Reflect on and share one's strengths and areas for improvement

Peers and Other Healthcare Providers

Consistent with principles of onboarding, social interactions play a huge role in the success of a new employee. Although the manager, educator, preceptor(s), and orientee may compose the group of key stakeholders, other healthcare providers (and especially their nurse peers) also play a role in successful orientation and onboarding of a new hire.

The role of others may include:

- Introducing self to orientee and getting to know him/her (even inviting him/her to social events will be helpful from an onboarding perspective)
- Providing the orientee a learning opportunity with one's patient assignment if the orientee needs that experience
- Giving feedback to preceptor(s) if the peer recognizes a strength or area for improvement

Conclusion

Assessing or evaluating competency is a huge undertaking due to its complexity; however, it is also the most pivotal moment in the orientation and onboarding process, as it will determine when an orientee can practice independently. If you use the AACN Synergy Model and Benner's competence continuum and layer your organization's definition of competence, you will have a robust understanding of what it takes to be successful.

For a nice example of one organization's approach to including many of the aforementioned models, check out Chapter 8, where we have included the form that Cincinnati Children's Hospital Medical Center has developed. Their model has been designed using the theoretical underpinnings of Benner's "Novice to Expert" model, the AACN Synergy Model, and the organization's job standards and clinical ladder.

Questions for Reflection/Discussion

1. Which approach to orientation (time-based or competency-based) do you see as being optimal, and why? How could your organization transition approaches if desired?

2. What does "competence" or "success" look like in your organization? To what degree are orientees made aware of what they need to do to be successful?

3. Where do you see many orientees having the greatest learning curve: cognitive knowledge, psychomotor skills, affective thoughts/behaviors, interpersonal skills, or critical thinking? Is there anything you could change about your orientation program to assist with this?

4. Which stakeholders in your organization have the most involvement in an orientee's training and evaluation? Should those who have the least involvement become more involved, and is there anything they could learn from those who have the most involvement?

KEY TAKEAWAYS

- *Competency-based orientation programs ensure that orientees are competent and haven't just spent the right amount of time in orientation and onboarding.*

- *Evaluating competency is a multi-faceted process.*

- *Competency assessment should consider cognitive knowledge, psychomotor skills, and affective thoughts and behaviors.*

- *Ensure key stakeholders play active roles in evaluating competency.*

References

Akerjordet, K., & Severinsson, E. (2007). Emotional intelligence: A review of the literature with a specific focus on empirical and epistemological perspectives. *Journal of Clinical Nursing, 16*(8), 1405–1416.

American Association of Colleges of Nursing (AACN). (2013). *Competencies and curricular expectations for Clinical Nurse Leader education and practice.* Retrieved from http://www.aacn.nche.edu/CNL

Anker, G. M. (2011). *Delmar's case study series: Medical-surgical nursing* (2nd ed.). Clifton Park, NY: Delmar.

Aradilla-Herrero, A., Tomás-Sábado, J., & Gómez-Benito, J. (2014). Perceived emotional intelligence in nursing: Psychometric properties of the Trait Meta-Mood Scale. *Journal of Clinical Nursing, 23*(7–8), 955–966.

Benner, P. (1982). From novice to expert. *The American Journal of Nursing, 82*(3), 402–407.

Freshwater, D., & Stickley, T. (2004). The heart of the art: Emotional intelligence in nurse education. *Nursing Inquiry, 11*(2), 91–98.

Goleman, D. (2006). *emotional intelligence: Why it can matter more than IQ* (10th Anniversary ed.). New York, NY: Bantam.

Harding, M., & Snyder, J. S. (2016). *Winningham's critical thinking cases in nursing: Medical-surgical, pediatric, maternity, and psychiatric* (6th ed.). St. Louis, MO: Mosby.

Insight Assessment. (2013). Health sciences reasoning test. Retrieved from http://www.insightassessment.com

Lunney, M. (2009). *Critical thinking to achieve positive health outcomes: Nursing case studies and analyses* (2nd ed.). Ames, IA: Wiley Blackwell.

McQueen, A. C. H. (2004). Emotional intelligence in nursing work. *Journal of Advanced Nursing, 47*(1), 101–108.

Melander, S. D. (2004). *Case studies in critical care nursing: A guide for application and review* (3rd ed.). Philadelphia, PA: Saunders.

Powell, K. R., Mabry, J. L., & Mixer, S. J. (2015). Emotional intelligence: A critical evaluation of the literature with implications for mental health nursing leadership. *Issues in Mental Health Nursing, 36*(5), 346–356.

Ulrich, B. (2011). *Mastering precepting: A nurse's handbook for success*. Indianapolis, IN: Sigma Theta Tau International.

CHAPTER 5

Working With Orientees

Introduction

Orientees will come to you with a wide variety of experiences, both personally and professionally, and the approach you take to working with them may vary just as much. Although the outcome of orientation should be the same for all nurses on the unit (providing safe and competent care), how the orientee travels through orientation may be unique. This chapter will focus on how to manage a variety of common orientee scenarios and help you develop strategies for working with them.

If you're short on time, you're welcome to jump to the page that discusses your particular situation. Are you working with an orientee who:

- Is a new graduate nurse? (p. 106)

- Is an experienced nurse? (p. 109)

- Is progressing quickly? (p. 110)

- Made an error? (p. 113)

- Has a personality conflict with his/her preceptor? (p. 115)

- Has a learning style that doesn't match his/her preceptor's teaching style? (p. 117)

- Struggles with interpersonal communication? (p. 118)

- Wants to quit? (p. 121)

- Can't successfully complete orientation? (p. 123)

Starting anything new is scary and overwhelming, much like when we all started our first day as a nurse. Energy high…hopeful to be a success…unbelievably proud of our new RN acronym…scared to hurt someone…terrified to look inadequate…needing to fit in and belong in this new group of coworkers…and astutely aware of how much there still is to learn.

Amy came to a point in her career that she had forgotten most of what *firsts* were like and had become more settled in feeling like the coworker these new nurses wanted to fit in with. She recounts her experience here:

> *"It was a point in my career I had felt I earned. I struggled and fought to grow and push myself. It was why I was called on to teach the newly onboarded staff. Instead of being empathetic, I exerted myself as the strong, silent type. I adopted the way of never let them see how really hard it is because they won't stay, and if they don't stay, I don't go on vacation. I wouldn't ever get to stop taking care of the hardest assignment, and mostly I have to deal with more from the next group of newbies who I may not like as much as the last.*
>
> *"I was wrong to look at the process that way. It really wasn't fair to those working so hard to gain knowledge I already had. I think after I realized this, I became a better teacher. I became empathetic versus situationally sympathetic. I shared their experiences, and I benefited from my preceptors who showed patience, kindness in less than perfect work, and the flexibility to teach me in the way that worked best for me. Was it fair to not be better when I knew better? My answer was 'no.' I had struggled too much in school to not really emotionally invest in the growth of those whom I taught. After all, doing a good job in nursing isn't just about tasks, understanding book knowledge, or checking off a checklist. It is about connection in our patients' darkest times. It is about existing in a place where vulnerability, sadness, hope, devastation, and grief live full time. That is not taught by a rigid, unrelatable taskmaster for a preceptor."*

Consider your first day at a job you hoped you would love for a long time. How many sights and sounds did you experience? How many times in that onboarding process did you hear, "Welcome! We are glad you are here!" and "This is a great place to work!"? What were the things that were done well, and what were the things that could be done better? Now it is your turn to get it right and struggle with the process. Empathy is an incredible tool for building relationships. It helps us connect with the hands-on work of nursing. If someone making important onboarding decisions doesn't keep in mind the essence of frontline staff's daily routines, how can we build an effective program?

While building orientation programs, keep in mind the view of the orientee and those staff working with an orientee. The tone begins with the staff educator. If staff is given clear expectations and goals, it is easy to see which orientees are meeting standards and which orientees aren't keeping pace. It also helps guide new preceptors in what to look for or to expect while teaching. If each orientee comes with a set of goals that primary preceptors make, anyone will be able to tell when the orientee needs more help or is meeting expectations.

Amy also shared, "I started becoming a better teacher by first figuring out how I would judge myself as a teacher. I decided to turn my focus away from my patient, and now the orientee became my new patient. It was tough. The work multiplied. I knew I wasn't patient enough, and I knew that I expected the new nurse to get it right the first time. The most important thing was to keep it simple. The orientee needs repetition, patience, freedom to learn from their mistakes in a non-judgmental environment, protection from big mistakes, and someone who can stand up for them when they can't stand up for themselves. I have made a million mistakes in precepting. Expecting too much too soon, being impatient saying, 'I already taught you that,' or 'How many times do I have to say it?' When a mistake happened, feeling ashamed of my orientee, feeling like my orientees' questions mean that I had failed as a teacher, and letting my orientee 'drown' without any emotional support were some of the pitfalls I fell into as a new preceptor. I began to form strategies of how to teach in an effective way that helped me pull out the best in each of the nurses I encountered."

We want to share Amy's strategies with you in the form of "preceptor pointers" embedded within several of the orientee case studies presented next. There are also a few general strategies at the end of the chapter. We believe these tips are essential for staff educators to apply and share with preceptors.

The New Graduate Nurse

New graduate (NG) nurses are, by far, the most predictable in their journeys. Even though their clinical and academic preparation may vary, they do not enter the professional realm with their own independent nursing experience upon which they can make decisions. They are like moldable clay that can be transformed into whatever you and your unit desire. Hopefully, that is both exciting and a little bit scary to you!

REAL-WORLD EXAMPLE: MOLDABLE MOLLY

Molly just started as an NG nurse on the unit. She is excited about being a nurse, but she is quite nervous about coming into work every day. Molly's preceptors have no concerns about her performance.

Molly goes to her educator and manager frequently with reports of, "I feel like I'm not getting it. I'm too slow, and I think I'm missing things. Everything seems so easy to my preceptor, and I've noticed that my friends are getting done with tasks faster than I am."

Molly is the typical NG nurse. She has enthusiasm and excitement while meeting the expectations of her preceptors. However, her confidence level is low. A nurse whose competence is on target but confidence is low requires encouragement, support, listening, and guided reflection. Provide frequent positive comments and focus on their strengths and the areas in which they have demonstrated great improvement. Listen to their concerns and let them know confidence is one of the last feelings an NG nurse acquires. Providing opportunities for reflection (both through in-person dialogue and journaling) will help them move more efficiently toward healthy self-confidence.

Encourage them not to compare themselves to their peers. They probably don't see how much their peers are actually doing, and everyone grows at different speeds based on the learning activities and patient experiences to which they are exposed. Reiterate that if concerns arise, you will let them know immediately. They typically are very open to feedback at this point, so don't hold anything back from them. Most likely, if you've heard it's a problem, they were probably wondering about it themselves.

Table 5.1 shows some of the behaviors you might see from an NG orientee and the appropriate responses to make.

TABLE 5.1 Behaviors and Responses for NG Orientees

BEHAVIORS	RESPONSES
Moldable Molly	Cheerleading Charlie
Excited/enthusiastic	Share in enthusiasm
Steadily increasing competence	Focus on growth and reaffirm strengths
Low confidence (scared of making an error)	Highlight performance so far
Compares self to peers	Discourage comparing self to others
Desires frequent feedback	Provide frequent and specific feedback (see Chapter 1 for feedback model)

Academic Preparation

Although most NG nurses are fairly similar in their lack of experience, there is one thing that might divide them further—their academic degree. Nurses can now enter the workforce with three different degrees: ADN, BSN, and MSN. Even though they all take the same licensure exam, the depth and breadth of certain professional nursing focus areas in their respective academic programs vary. Briefly, here are some differences that Alvin has noticed in their orientation.

Associate's Degree in Nursing (ADN)

Nurses with an ADN likely will have received less theoretical and abstract courses in their curriculum. Because their primary focus has been placed on clinical components, you may see that their clinical skills are acquired more quickly than their peers with other degrees. On the other hand, they may require more assistance from the organization with participating in larger improvement/change projects and systematically integrating research and evidence into their practice.

Bachelor of Science in Nursing (BSN)

Nurses with a BSN will have had a balanced preparation in both clinical and theoretical components of nursing practice. Many acute care hospitals now require a BSN for NG nurses; therefore, if you work in one of those organizations, the majority of your new hires will hold a BSN, and your orientation program should be focused on this majority. BSN-prepared NG nurses likely will need more support in their clinical skills and critical thinking rather than helping them to wrap their heads around rationales for unit-level change projects and the importance of changing practice to reflect current evidence.

Master of Science in Nursing (MSN)

Nurses who enter the profession with an MSN as their initial nursing degree should have a similar clinical preparation as their BSN counterparts, but there is so much focus on leadership and systems thinking that this may overshadow their clinical competence initially. While these NG nurses should be encouraged to think outside the box and get involved in department and organizational projects, they may need to be redirected to focus on clinical skills during their initial orientation to professional nursing. They may require more frequent reminders about placing emphasis on day-to-day activities until those have been mastered. However, once these patient care skills have been mastered, MSN-prepared nurses should be well-poised to quickly grow into leadership roles.

Nurse Residency Programs

Nurse residency programs have increased in both quantity and quality in recent years, and their utility has been proven (Krugman et al., 2006; Pine & Tart, 2007) in many organizations. These programs have assisted NG nurses in quickly transitioning to their role as professional nurses while also drastically reducing first-year turnover. Some hospitals are beginning to provide modified residency programs for newly hired nurses who have previous nursing experience with another organization. Check out the "Nurse Residency Programs" section of Chapter 3 for additional resources.

The Experienced Nurse

Experienced nurses are those nurses who have had at least 9 to 12 months of providing patient care outside of their academic training. Experience can span a wide variety of years as well as specialties, and although an experienced nurse has established the foundations of critical thinking (and hopefully psychomotor skill), moving to a new specialty can be overwhelming. The greater the change in specialty, the more difficult the transition may be (e.g., transitioning from adult hospice to pediatric critical care will be a larger change than transitioning from a medical intensive care unit to a surgical intensive care unit).

REAL-WORLD EXAMPLE: EXPERIENCED ELEANOR

Eleanor has 5 years of experience working with telemetry patients in an adult hospital. She has decided that she would like to work with children, so she has taken a job in a neonatal intensive care unit.

Eleanor's preceptors note that she is slow to document and respond to patient alarms, but there are no issues with medication administration or patient assessments. Eleanor tells her educator and manager, "The babies are just so much smaller than I'm used to. I have no problem giving out the medications, but my preceptor keeps telling me I'm not prioritizing correctly."

Your role in staff development will be to help the orientee (and the preceptor) identify knowledge gaps and learning opportunities to bridge those gaps. Whether those opportunities are classes, self-directed reading and studying, or patient assignments, selecting the best learning activities for an experienced nurse will be key in his/her success. Chances are high that if the experienced nurse was successful in a previous organization or department, he/she will be successful in yours, given the appropriate guidance and learning opportunities.

If you are working with preceptors who are more familiar with NG nurses, the preceptors may need to be reminded that experienced nurses develop differently than NG nurses because they have experiences that have shaped their approach to patient care and decision-making. If decision-making (regarding things such as time management and prioritization) needs to occur differently than it did in their previous environment, the preceptor will need to identify these differences and attempt to verbalize what may be unspoken or implicit knowledge among nurses in the department. For example, the preceptors should verbally state, "If you're short on time, the medical team would like to see vital signs and physical assessment charted before intake and output," or "Don't put your whole lunch box in the refrigerator because if everyone does that on day shift, it takes up too much space. Try to place only cold items in there."

PRECEPTOR POINTER: THERE IS NO RIGHT WAY

There is no right way—there is simply safe and congruent with policy. Let's do it my way first because I know it is safe and congruent with policy because I understand it. Then build your own way that you know is safe and congruent with policy because you understand it.

Consult Table 5.2 for some of the behaviors you might see from an experienced nurse orientee and appropriate actions you can take.

TABLE 5.2 Behaviors and Responses for Experienced Nurse Orientees

BEHAVIORS	RESPONSES
Experienced Eleanor	Guiding Gail
Basic nursing skills mastered & specialty nursing skills quickly acquired	Assist orientee in integrating these basic and specialty skills
Uses previous experiences/methods for managing time & priorities	Verbalize implicit/unspoken behaviors and group thought processes

The Quickly Progressing Nurse

Some nurses will progress through orientation more quickly than the average new hire. For NG nurses this can be a result of receiving greater academic and/or clinical preparation, entering the workplace with more life experience, or having an increased capacity for cognitive and/or emotional intelligence. For experienced nurses, a quicker progression will more likely occur if their previous environment is similar to the new one.

REAL-WORLD EXAMPLE: QUICK QUINTON

Quinton is a new graduate orientee in an outpatient orthopedic clinic who is well liked and respected by current staff, including the surgeons and management. Quinton tells his educator, "I'm feeling good about things, and I really like it here."

REAL-WORLD EXAMPLE: AVERAGE ALLIE

Allie is also a new graduate who started with Quinton, and she is right on track with completing orientation in the expected time allotment. There are no issues with her performance, but she tends to be shy in social settings and doesn't personally know the staff as well as Quinton does. Allie repeatedly says to her preceptor, "I'm just not getting it. It's all too much for me, and I don't feel like I'm doing anything right. Maybe this place isn't for me."

Once the quickly progressing orientee builds a reputation for "catching on quickly," the preceptors and peers may assume he/she knows more than he/she actually does. Although it is important to acknowledge progression and competency, learning is a never-ending process in healthcare, and there is always additional information which the new hire could benefit from learning. Staff development specialists should remind preceptors not to decrease their rigor while evaluating continued progress. Preceptors may need additional training in how to verbally structure their teaching moments in such a way that acknowledges the new hire's proficiency while simultaneously offering potentially new or forgotten information. For example, instead of asking, "Have you done [insert skill] before?" it may be better to ask, "What has been your experience with [insert skill]?" This allows for a wider variety of responses rather than simply a "yes/no."

If several new hires start orientation at the same time (such as a cohort), some may begin to feel their performance is inadequate compared to the quickly progressing orientee. This is most notable with NG cohorts and needs to be handled delicately. Requiring significantly more positive reinforcement than their experienced counterparts, NG nurses frequently compare themselves with the other peers in their cohort to self-assess their progress. When they see other orientees progressing more quickly or finishing orientation earlier, the average- or slower-progressing orientee may have profound episodes of self-doubt and begin to frequently ask what is wrong with their practice.

PRECEPTOR POINTER: SUPERVISION

For quickly progressing orientees: I will stand by you for every task until I have confidence you can achieve that task successfully. Once that is true, you get some space, and it is your job to signal me when you need more help than I am providing.

For slower progressing orientees: You can't take on the whole of it today, so what piece of the pie can we tackle? I (preceptor) am responsible for the whole pie. You will be responsible one day when you are ready.

Tables 5.3 and 5.4 cover some behaviors and appropriate responses when you are dealing both with quickly progressing orientees and their peers, who might be progressing at a slower, albeit normal, pace.

TABLE 5.3 Behaviors and Responses for Quickly Progressing Orientees

BEHAVIORS	RESPONSES
Quick Quinton	Consistent Connie
Reaches milestones ahead of time	Recognize accomplishments
Well-liked by other staff	Encourage continued socialization/ onboarding
Labeled as an "easy orientee" by preceptor	Maintain consistent, rigorous evaluation standards equivalent to other orientees
	Ask open-ended questions that acknowledge expertise while also creating a potential learning opportunity

TABLE 5.4
Behaviors and Responses for the Peers of Quickly Progressing Orientees

BEHAVIORS	RESPONSES
Average Allie	Re-Focusing Riley
No performance issues	Reaffirm strengths
Frequently questions self-progress	Focus on growth
Mentions peers' actions more than her own	Redirect attention to orientee's performance

When Orientees Make Errors

All healthcare providers, regardless of profession, specialty, and experience level, are at risk for making errors. Just as the title of the Institute of Medicine (2000) report so appropriately stated, *To Err Is Human*. Making an error may become even easier when a clinician is exposed to a new environment that requires a new set of competencies. Therefore, errors are not uncommon during the orientation period, and you need to balance the normalcy of making errors with the excellent learning opportunity they present.

REAL-WORLD EXAMPLE: MED MIX-UP MELANIE

Melanie is a new nurse in a long-term care facility in which the rooms are designed such that two patients can be present in the same room. Melanie was administering medications one morning before breakfast to two patients who required different doses of insulin, and she administered the wrong dose to both of them.

The patient who received too much insulin collapsed to the floor when getting up to use the restroom. The patient quickly regained consciousness and was placed back in bed where her glucose was normalized with oral, sugar-containing fluids. She had no long-term injuries.

Errors can occur in a wide variety of situations, and their impact severity can range from near-miss to death. The approach to working with an orientee who has made an error will be largely influenced by the scope and impact of the error.

In Melanie's case, the error resulted in temporary harm to the patient. If Melanie were a new graduate (or experienced but with little confidence at this point), this error could be devastating to her self-confidence. Therefore, the preceptor (as well as other supporting players such as the staff development specialist, manager, peers, etc.) needs to assess the orientee's feelings of the situation. You can start by using Gibbs's reflective cycle (see Figure 5.1) and accompanying questions (Gibbs, 1988). Depending on the orientee's reaction to the situation, the supporting persons may need to help Melanie focus on the involvement of various systems factors (such as room design, the medication administration process, etc.) in the error occurrence. This can help Melanie understand how anyone can be prone to errors.

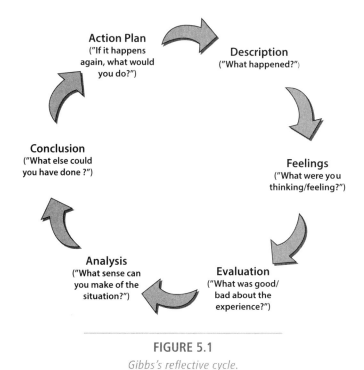

FIGURE 5.1

Gibbs's reflective cycle.

If the error resulted in more severe harm to the patient, professional counseling may be required, and the organization should provide assistance in receiving this support. Conversely, if the error did not reach the patient (a near-miss), the preceptor should seek to determine if the orientee understands the impact this "close call" could have had.

Regardless of the impact on confidence, the error should always be used as a learning opportunity. Many newer nurses will cope with the situation by developing a mentality that will make them hyperaware of the precipitating factors in the future. Some paraphrase this mindset by stating, "Well, I know I will never do that again!"

Finally, all errors, including near-misses, should be communicated to the appropriate risk-management personnel in the organization, who can look into preventing this from happening in the future.

> **PRECEPTOR POINTER: HEARING FEEDBACK**
>
> *Tell the orientee (and yourself): "You will not get it right the first time, so being hard on yourself only slows your ability to try again. If you bring a good attitude with you each time we step to a task, we will get it right eventually."*

Table 5.5 suggests appropriate responses to keep in mind when orientees make errors.

TABLE 5.5 Behaviors and Responses for Orientees Who Make an Error

BEHAVIORS	RESPONSES
Med Mix-Up Melanie	Comforting & Clarifying Cathy
Preoccupied with the error	Care for patient immediately after event
Decreased confidence	Comfort orientee
Concerned about making the same mistake again	Discuss strategies for doing it correctly

Personality Conflicts

Regardless of the skill and expertise of the assigned preceptor, personality conflicts are bound to arise during the orientation period. Orientees and preceptors can vary in their experience level, educational background, gender, race, culture, values, and social norms. Although nurses may possess great skill in taking care of patients who differ from them, it can become quite stressful for a preceptor to balance care for patients while also working with a new hire. This may be comparable to taking on two sets of patients concurrently. Additionally, the orientees are under a high degree of stress simply because of the massive learning trajectory they face.

When these stressors are placed in the context of a complex healthcare environment, it may be difficult to adapt and "keep your cool" when faced with what appears to be an impossible task. The capacity to be empathetic and patient is diminished in these situations, and incompatible personalities in the teacher-learner dyad further complicate the problem.

REAL-WORLD EXAMPLE: PERSONALITY PROBLEM PAULA

Paula is a new graduate nurse in a psychiatric hospital whose preceptor, Alan, is very concerned that "she just isn't getting it." The staff development specialist has met with Paula and feels that she isn't progressing as quickly as she should be but is fairly confident she has the knowledge and skills needed to be successful.

Alan has been caught raising his voice at Paula and even slapping her hand as Paula is about to perform a small task incorrectly. Both Paula and Alan get very frustrated when their patient assignment is busy or when high acuity situations occur. Paula states, "Alan is just so mean and doesn't teach me anything beneficial. I don't think he likes me."

Ideally, preceptors and orientees should be paired by complementary personality styles, if known. This could be achieved by soliciting input from someone who personally knows both of them, or by using select personality tools (e.g., the Myers-Briggs Type Indicator [MBTI] or DISC, which are found in Chapter 2).

If it is not possible to match (either due to not knowing the orientee or not having a large enough preceptor pool) or if this matching was not successful, additional assessments should be performed to uncover the cause of the conflicting personalities. The preceptor and orientee need to verbalize their natural tendencies regarding communication and decision-making and open the conversation to discuss these differences. This is one of those "easier said than done" activities that may benefit from having a mediator present, such as a staff development specialist.

The staff development specialist should bring the preceptor and the orientee together in a quiet meeting space. The purpose of the meeting is to help create a proper line of communication. Questions to use for the meeting include:

- How do you like to give feedback? Receive feedback?
- How do you like to receive praise? Constructive criticism?
- What is your favorite thing about your job?
- What is your least favorite thing about your job?
- What are your pet peeves and/or hot buttons?
- What ground rules would you propose to keep the lines of communication open with this other person?

The staff development specialist can give them some silent time for each to make notes about his/her response to the questions, and then the specialist would facilitate a discussion about their answers and get them to agree to ground rules moving forward.

If none of these interventions resolve the problem, it may be necessary to assign the orientee to a different preceptor. Managers and educators should reinforce to the preceptor that irreconcilable differences do occur, and successful orientation of the new hire is the priority. However, this may also be an opportunity for professional development of the preceptor, and after assessing his/her behaviors and communication styles, he/she may learn new approaches for working with orientees in the future.

Alvin's experience has been that preceptors initially may be upset by the decision to place their orientees with someone else. However, those preceptors are frequently thankful for that decision by the end of the new hire's orientation period, once they see the various challenges the new preceptor-orientee pair faced.

Table 5.6 can help you spot the behaviors and respond appropriately when preceptors and orientees have personality conflicts.

TABLE 5.6
Behaviors and Responses for Orientees Who Have a Personality Conflict With a Preceptor

BEHAVIORS	RESPONSES
Personality Problem Paula	Adaptable Alan
Easily frustrated	Display patience
Not receptive to feedback	Investigate orientee's preferred method for learning and receiving feedback
Speaks poorly of preceptor to others	
	Verbalize desire for orientee's success

Teaching/Learning Style Conflicts

Many of the concepts found in working with personality conflicts also hold true with teaching/learning style conflicts. In fact, it can be difficult, initially, to determine if the frustrations of a preceptor and/

or orientee are due to a true personality conflict or, more simply, if the orientee has a learning style the preceptor is not considering when teaching.

As in personality conflict, the most ideal situation is to match preceptors and orientees with similar learning styles. If the preceptor has a similar learning style, he/she is more likely to teach in a way that is easily received by the orientee. Several available tools can assess learning styles, including but not limited to: Kolb, MBTI, and Visual/Auditory/Reading-Writing/Kinesthetic (see Chapter 2 for more information).

If pairing similar learning styles is not possible, preceptor development and training can prove very beneficial. By helping the preceptor to modify his/her preferred teaching style based on the orientee's learning style, orientees will acquire the necessary knowledge and skills in a shorter period of time and (hopefully) with less frustration for both.

For preceptors who have not had formal training in education strategies, it can be easy to assume that all people learn in a similar manner as they do. Alvin has frequently heard nurses say, "We learn by being hands-on, not by reading it or hearing about it." Although the majority of nurses may be sensory, and even more specifically, kinesthetic learners (Frankel, 2009; Smith, 2010), not all nurses can be placed into this category, and effective preceptors will adapt their teaching styles to their orientees' learning styles.

Struggling With Interpersonal Communication

Although nurses receive training on skillful and therapeutic communication during their academic preparation, activities such as active listening and carefully selecting the right words to say may be more difficult to apply when communicating with a coworker rather than a patient. The peer-peer and preceptor-orientee relationships can be quite different from the nurse-patient relationship. Workplace relationships are longer lasting, and nurses' capacity for patience and empathy may not be as great toward their peers. This can be complicated by unit/department culture and social norms, many of which will be new to an orientee.

REAL-WORLD EXAMPLE: DEFENSIVE DAN

Dan is an experienced nurse who recently transferred to the trauma-surgical intensive care unit from a medical intensive care unit in a nearby hospital. When his preceptor attempts to provide feedback about his performance, Dan regularly responds harshly, and he has been known to simply walk away.

Dan tells his educator, "I don't think people like me here. It's like people don't want me to do well here, and they always are criticizing me." As the educator performs follow-up, discussions with the preceptor, Gina, reveal it can be very challenging for Gina to give Dan feedback about his performance and that Dan is resistant to being taught skills that are performed differently from his previous institution.

Many of the concepts discussed in the personality conflict section apply to this situation, too. In fact, it can be difficult to differentiate between personality conflicts and communication struggles because a person's communication style can be influenced by his/her temperament and character. The most important component of managing interpersonal communication challenges in the preceptor-orientee relationship will be to discuss openly the expectations of both parties. This may involve answering questions like:

- When does the orientee prefer to receive feedback (e.g., in real time or at the end of the shift)?
- Where should feedback be provided (e.g., in the patient's room, at the nurse's station, or in a break room)?
- How will expectations for the day (or week) be established and evaluated?
- How much involvement does the orientee expect from the preceptor?

While this conversation can be mediated by a third party if requested, honestly discussing expectations and mutually agreeing upon acceptable behaviors will be fundamental to create an environment in which the orientee has the optimal learning opportunity.

Most interpersonal communication struggles will occur between healthcare providers; however, some new hires may struggle in communicating with patients and families. Hopefully, this was identified and addressed during the academic program. However, the stresses of a new work environment may make it difficult for a new hire to communicate appropriately with patients and families. If this is the case, the orientee should first be told that patients and families perceive his/her communication as inappropriate or difficult to understand. Many times, simply stating this perception will be enough for the new hire to admit to an elevated stress level, which then opens the discussion for establishing healthy coping mechanisms and, eventually, effective communication strategies.

PRECEPTOR POINTER: HEARING FEEDBACK

I will tell you how to improve—it will be hard to hear because we are going to talk about the good and the bad. If you need to step away to process or take a break, do it. The responsibility in this work is hard, and knowing your limits and boundaries to bring your best is essential. Some days it will be easy to hear how you need to improve, and some days it will be quite difficult. It is part of the growing process.

For an orientee who does not see a need to change his/her communication style, the manager should quickly be brought into the discussion to determine if the employee's skill set and professional goals are a good match for the organization's mission and vision. If an incongruence surfaces, you may want to jump to the section "Orientees unable to Successfully Complete Orientation" later in the chapter.

Table 5.7 shows the signs of an orientee having communication struggles and suggests what you can do about it.

TABLE 5.7
Behaviors and Responses for Orientees Who Struggle with Interpersonal Communication

BEHAVIORS	RESPONSES
Defensive Dan	Gentle Gina
May not be receptive to feedback	Investigate orientee's preferred method for learning and receiving feedback
Quick- or hot-tempered at times	
	Display patience
Verbalizes feelings of "not fitting in"	
	Facilitate socialization by engaging both orientee and peers
Doesn't engage in socialization opportunities	

Wanting to Quit

Some literature suggests the percentage of new graduate nurses who choose to leave their first job within their first year is as great as 60% (Godinez, Schweiger, Gruver, & Ryan, 1999). Ideally, implementing recommendations from this book and other sources will help you and your organization keep your first-year turnover rate far below this mark. However, even under ideal situations with optimal work environments and healthy interpersonal relationships, some new hires may simply not enjoy the specific patient population for whom your department provides nursing care.

REAL-WORLD EXAMPLE: DISINTERESTED DEREK

Derek started working in the surgical intensive care unit of a large urban medical center as a new graduate nurse. He previously worked in the unit as an administrative assistant during nursing school, and he did many clinical experiences in the neighboring medical intensive care unit. During nursing school, he frequently questioned whether or not he wanted to work in the unit as a nurse. He executed his administrative assistant duties with superb ratings, and his coworkers convinced him that he should pursue a nursing position after graduation.

During orientation, Derek acquired his skills quickly and got along well with his preceptor. However, he struggled a bit with confidence and continued to question whether or not this was the right place for him. Toward the end of orientation, after being exposed to a wide variety of patient experiences, he verbalized to his manager, "I just don't think this place is for me. I didn't realize how sick these patients can get, and I don't think I like my patients being this ill."

Begin your assessment of the situation with ensuring that the orientee truly dislikes the patient population as opposed to some other aspect of the work environment, or conflicts or issues such as those mentioned in previous sections of this chapter. Pending no other identified problems, working with an orientee who simply does not find fulfillment (or outright hates) caring for the patient population in your area can be a challenge.

Ideally, the hiring process ensures candidates who are not truly passionate about the selected patient population are not hired. However, even the best talent-acquisition processes may allow some candidates through the cracks. This is especially true of new graduate orientees who may not know what their desired patient population is yet.

Once this desire to leave is confirmed, guidance from Human Resources may be needed to assist with the next steps. Some organizations do not allow new hires to transfer to another department within their probationary period. Because it is likely that the probationary period cannot be completed until orientation is wrapped up, the orientee may have to successfully complete orientation and begin caring for patients in your department until their probationary period is done.

Additionally, transferring within the organization early in one's career may look suspicious to the department to which the new hire is applying to work. The staff development specialist and/or manager can assist with this transition by writing a letter of recommendation, commenting on the orientee's proficiency in caring for the patient population, and explaining the situation, if the orientee requests such a letter. (Please check with Human Resources before writing recommendation letters for other employees to ensure compliance with organizational guidelines.)

Finally, preceptors should be reassured that the orientee's desire to leave is in no way a reflection of the preceptor's performance but rather a personal choice to work with a different patient population.

PRECEPTOR POINTER: CHECKING IN

I will check in often to ask if you are OK and if what we are doing together is helping. I need to hear the honest truth. It slows your progress for you to shrug it off and just say you are fine when you are not. It doesn't allow me to help you or you to help yourself.

Consult Table 5.8 to prepare yourself for behaviors you might see from orientees who want to quit and to ready yourself to respond.

TABLE 5.8 Behaviors and Responses for Orientees Who Want to Quit

BEHAVIORS	RESPONSES
Disinterested Derek	Understanding Ursula
No performance issues	Reaffirm strengths
High stress level and/or low confidence	Emphasize orientee's positive impact on patient/family
Verbalizes desire to quit	
	Listen and assist with decision-making

Orientees Unable to Successfully Complete Orientation

Probably the most challenging and least desirable of all orientation situations is when a new hire is unable to successfully complete orientation. Even though all nurses complete comparable academic studies and pass the same national licensure exam, not every individual's combination of knowledge, skills, attitudes, and decision-making styles is appropriate for the patient population and/or organization with whom he/she chooses to work.

REAL-WORLD EXAMPLE: STRUGGLING STACI

Staci is a new graduate nurse in the operating room whom all the staff adore. She is kind to all patients and peers, and she communicates effectively. However, multiple safety incidents have resulted from her performance, including many near-misses and even a couple events that resulted in temporary harm to the patient. All of these events were reviewed with her, and additional training was provided. Yet, some behaviors resulted in repeated events.

Staci tells her educator, "I promise I'm trying because I really do want to work here. I just don't understand how all of this keeps happening." Staci is tearful during these conversations.

For the nurses serving as the preceptors, managers, and staff development specialists, one of the most difficult challenges is listening to more than the caring and compassionate voice inside you that says, "But she's really sweet. She might eventually get it." As nurses, we possess a great ability for seeing and appreciating the value of every human being. Although this skill is necessary in caring for patients, it can make it difficult for us to objectively evaluate peers or colleagues.

Early signs of inadequate performance may be noticed at the beginning of orientation, but it will likely take some time to determine that an employee may need to be terminated. No new hire enters the organization without the need for at least some training and orientation, but some employees will reach a point at which additional training will not provide sufficient assistance for them to work independently in a safe and effective manner.

Identifying the point at which training will no longer be beneficial is complicated. Some organizations have a standard length of orientation, and orientees who cannot complete orientation within that designated time are terminated. Other organizations have a competency-based approach, and the educator and manager may have to rely on the average of previous new hires' orientation time to decide when the process is taking too long.

When you are concerned that an orientee may not be able to successfully complete orientation, you should try to determine the factors preventing him/her from being successful (which are hopefully discussed earlier in this chapter) and alleviate those problems. Manager involvement should be solicited at the moment you are concerned, because if all efforts to improve performance prove unsuccessful, it will be the manager's responsibility to coordinate the termination process. Check out Chapter 8 for suggestions on how to work collaboratively with your Human Resources department.

Regardless of the process and speed of termination, the preceptor should continue to focus on incorporating strategies mentioned elsewhere in this text in an attempt to correct or improve performance issues. These continued efforts to provide a successful orientation experience may eventually give the orientee what he/she needs to "turn the corner" and maintain employment. In all circumstances, however, detailed documentation of preceptor efforts and orientee responses is essential.

Table 5.9 goes over the behaviors of orientees who can't successfully complete orientation and your possible responses to that situation.

TABLE 5.9
Behaviors and Responses for Orientees
Who Are Unable to Successfully Complete Orientation

BEHAVIORS	RESPONSES
Struggling Staci	Persistent Patrick
Significant performance issues but potentially unaware of them	Continue teaching and providing feedback
	Acknowledge orientee's efforts
Will likely verbalize desire to improve and may go "above and beyond" with some tasks to demonstrate competency	Document preceptor interventions and orientee behaviors in detail
May be easily frustrated with tasks	Maintain frequent communication with manager and/or educator

Conclusion

Orientees come in a wide variety of shapes and sizes, and the interventions required to transform them into safe and effective clinicians can be just as varied. Especially for those orientees who do not follow a "typical" pathway through orientation, identifying their challenges may not be as simple as represented in this chapter. Additionally, some orientees may fit somewhere in between these classifications and require pick-and-choose interventions from different categories. Whatever struggles arise, open communication and strong collaboration between all involved parties will be essential to the orientee's success.

Some additional Preceptor Pointers we believe can apply in almost all situations include the following.

PRECEPTOR POINTER:
SETTING GOALS AND EXPECTATIONS

Ask the questions. Ask them 100 times if you need to because the worst thing you can do is not understand why you are doing a task. When you ask orientees to blindly follow, they have to trust that you are doing it with the intention of eventually teaching them why.

"We will set two goals for our day. If we get more done, great! But limiting the large amount of things we need to get done is important for not overwhelming the learning process.

"We will stop learning new material at 2:00. From there on, we will just repeat. Repetition helps your brain process all the new material I have shared with you.

"I will not know the answer to every question, and neither will you. Let me show you how to use your resources to find the answers, and then I expect you to practice it over and over and over again."

Questions for Reflection/Discussion

1. What academic preparation do your typical new graduate nursing orientees have?

2. How prepared is your orientation program for new graduate nurses who do not have the typical academic preparation the rest of your orientees have?

3. Which of the listed orientee types is most prevalent in your unit, department, or organization?

4. Which of the listed orientee types would be easiest and most difficult for you (the professional development specialist) to manage? Why?

5. Which of the listed orientee types is most difficult for your staff members (direct care providers, preceptors, charge nurses, etc.) to work with? Why?

6. What preparation do your preceptors have to manage these various orientee types?

7. What preparation do your managers have to manage these various orientee types?

KEY TAKEAWAYS

- *Orientees come with a wide array of backgrounds, personalities, and characteristics, and your approach to working with them will vary just as much.*

- *There is not a "one size fits all" approach to any specific orientee consideration, but you will begin to see themes and patterns after you work with them long enough. Until then, try some of the approaches we have outlined in this chapter.*

- *Creating an orientation program that has an ample amount of flexibility will help to successfully accommodate a variety of orientees.*

- *Open lines of communication between the staff development specialist, the orientee, the preceptor, and the hiring manager are critical to the success of any onboarding process.*

References

Frankel, A. (2009, January 20). Nurses' learning styles: Promoting better integration of theory into practice. *Nursing Times, 105*(2), 24–27.

Gibbs, G. (1988). *Learning by doing: A guide to teaching and learning methods.* Oxford, England: Oxford Polytechnic.

Godinez, G., Schweiger, J., Gruver, J., & Ryan, P. (1999). Role transition from graduate to staff nurse: A qualitative analysis. *Journal for Nurses in Staff Development, 15*(3), 97–110.

Institute of Medicine (IOM). (2000). *To err is human: Building a safer health system.* Washington, DC: National Academies Press.

Krugman, M., Bretschneider, J., Horn, P. B., Krsek, C. A., Moutafis, R. A., & Smith, M. O. (2006). The national post-baccalaureate graduate nurse residency program: A model for excellence in transition to practice. *Journal for Nurses in Staff Development, 22*(4), 196–205.

Pine, R., & Tart, K. (2007). Return on investment: Benefits and challenges of a baccalaureate nurse residency program. *Nursing Economic$, 25*(1), 13–18, 39.

Smith, A. (2010). Learning styles of registered nurses enrolled in an online nursing program. *Journal of Professional Nursing, 26*(1), 49–53. doi: 10.1016/j.profnurs.2009.04.006

CHAPTER 6

Evaluating an Orientation Program

Introduction

Orientation programs, regardless of their design or structure, should be evaluated for their efficacy. Just as the nursing process and ADDIE model complete their cycles with Evaluation, so too, do all successful programs. By evaluating your orientation program from various perspectives and levels, you ensure an effective, efficient orientation program that adds value to the individual, the unit/department, and the organization—a win-win-win situation.

Evaluating an orientation program should provide you with useful information that will do one of two things:

1. Describe areas of the program that need to be modified because they are not as effective or efficient as they could be

2. Supply evidence that the program is in fact doing what it's supposed to do

Although this may sound simple and self-evident, consider the following two examples in which having documented, objective evaluation data proved useful.

REAL-WORLD EXAMPLE: THE NEED FOR EVALUATION #1

Dan was the staff development specialist in charge of the first week of nursing orientation for all new hires entering his organization. When he assumed this role, he discovered that evaluation of this first week of training was performed by a simple survey on the last day of the week which asked these new hires if they liked the content they learned. Although Dan knew this was a good start, he felt more should be done to evaluate his program. So, he developed a survey for preceptors to complete within the first 2 weeks a new hire spent on the unit taking care of patients. This survey evaluated basic skills observed by the preceptor.

Dan quickly discovered that documentation in the electronic medical record was a problem among new hires in most departments. Therefore, he modified the training day on documentation to include more case-based and simulation scenarios. Post-intervention data revealed improved documentation performance, and anecdotal feedback came to him from unit-based educators who said the new hires' ability to document efficiently had drastically increased preceptor satisfaction and allowed them to cover more advanced skills much earlier.

This example shows how including various levels of evaluation provides for a more well-rounded assessment of program efficacy and highlights potential opportunities for improvement.

REAL-WORLD EXAMPLE: THE NEED FOR EVALUATION #2

Marie, a unit-based educator, was invited to attend a meeting with other unit-based educators as well as several senior-level managers who had a strong influence on training and development in the organization. Due to economic hardships, the managers informed the educators that various "non-essential" components of initial orientation would be removed. Notably, an 8-hour class on medication safety was being removed from central orientation based on the rationale that licensed healthcare providers should already be familiar with this information, and preceptors should be reinforcing it at the unit level.

Although Marie had a "gut feeling" that this class should not be removed (and she knew that her own new hires found this class beneficial), she knew she would need more objective data to prevent the removal of the class. After the meeting, Marie gathered already-available data on rates of serious adverse drug events, starting with data collected approximately 2 years before the medication safety class was added to central orientation. Marie shared the data with managers and showed them how implementation of this class resulted in a 50% decrease of serious adverse drug events and saved the organization more money than what was spent on salary for attending the class. The managers decided to keep this class in orientation.

This example shows the value of collecting objective evaluation data for the purpose of maintaining orientation components that have proven value.

Alvin's experience in teaching project-management strategies to nurses has revealed that objectively evaluating a project or program does not come naturally for many nurses. Evaluation of a program (or even a change in a program) should stem from the assessment data that warranted its presence. Unfortunately, many nurses settle for a level of evaluation as simple as satisfaction with the program, even though the program was created due to a problem noted with patient care. These various levels of evaluation will be discussed throughout the chapter, but first we want to provide you with an example that will hopefully hit home.

We want to share this example as a way of showing the parallels between evaluating an orientation program and a patient's pain.

EVALUATING A PROGRAM IS LIKE EVALUATING A PATIENT'S PAIN

Consider the case of a 35-year-old patient with multiple rib fractures due to a motor vehicle accident. The patient is in pain because of the presence of a chest tube as well as movement of his ribs while breathing. He rates his pain as an 8 out of 10 on the numeric rating scale, and you (as the nurse) provide him with a standard, adult dose of intravenous morphine. Which of the following sets of questions would be most valuable for evaluating the effectiveness of the pain medication after administration?

QUESTION SET A	QUESTION SET B
On a scale of 0–10, how satisfied are you with my ability to administer a pain medication?	On a scale of 0–10, how would you rate your pain now?
Do you think your pain level has changed as a result of the administering of this medication?	Is the pain level you're experiencing now manageable?
Would you recommend this pain medication to other patients?	Do you need additional help in managing your pain?

Obviously, Question Set B is the appropriate response.

Nurses are phenomenal at assessing and reassessing pain, and they are focused on one major goal—keeping the patient as comfortable as possible. As the patient's pain increases, an intervention is carried out, and the nurse reassesses to ensure the pain has decreased. Similarly, if there is a performance issue in the organization, and a new component were added in orientation to address this performance issue, the best evaluation would involve assessing the continued presence of the performance issue (not whether new hires enjoyed the training or scored better on a test).

We're not trying to minimize the importance of evaluating satisfaction with an orientation program; however, we want you to realize that evaluating an orientation program should not stop at this first level. Appropriate evaluation will relate back to the assessment data that initially suggested the need for the intervention's creation. We hope you'll keep this in mind as you read this chapter.

Levels and Types of Evaluation

Several models are used in business and education for evaluating the efficacy of a program or project, but Kirkpatrick's Four Levels of Evaluation is probably the most notable and the one from which many other evaluation models originate.

Kirkpatrick's Four Levels of Evaluation

The reason for widespread use of Kirkpatrick's model is primarily due to the simplicity and practicality of his approach (Kirkpatrick, 1996). His four levels are: reaction, learning, behavior, and results. Pros and cons of each level are listed in Table 6.1, and you can see examples of how to apply each of these levels to actual programs in Table 6.2.

Reaction

The first level, reaction, deals with the learners' reaction to the training program (what their experience was like during the activity). Assessment of this level could include any aspect of the program from speaker, to content and environment, to delivery style. This level of evaluation provides insight into learner satisfaction. Many training and development professionals refer to this level of evaluation as "smiley sheets." As many of you are probably aware, if content isn't delivered in a way that makes it interesting to the learner, there is little chance that the learner will put forth any effort to absorb the information (Kirkpatrick, 1996).

The reaction level is commonly evaluated in training programs due to its ease of measurement and the ability to make quick changes based on feedback. It should be measured relatively soon after a program is delivered because participants may quickly forget things like how conducive the room was to learning.

Learning

The next level, learning, assesses how well knowledge is transferred to the learner. This could include learning in any of the cognitive, psychomotor, and even affective (attitude) domains (Kirkpatrick, 1996). While the first level asks participants for their perspective of the program, learning will be a more objective assessment that is typically measured through written tests and/or observation.

This level of evaluation is slightly more complex than the reaction level of evaluation, but it is still fairly simple to design and quite common in training programs. For example, anyone who has participated in a continuing education program online and taken a test at the end regarding the content has had their learning assessed. The best way to measure learning would be to provide pre- and post-program tests and calculate the difference between the two scores. Also, it is possible to assess learning through simulations and/or case studies.

Behavior

At this third level, evaluation begins to become much more difficult. Evaluating the level of behavior involves what Kirkpatrick (1996) refers to as transfer of training. To assess this level of evaluation, you must observe behavioral changes in the learner in their actual job setting. A challenge with this level is that you do not have control of what the learner encounters in the real-world setting.

For example, if you delivered a program on pressure ulcer reduction, you might want to observe whether or not nurses are turning patients at the appropriate frequency, as well as if they are properly using pressure-relieving equipment. If they are not, then you might want to see what is preventing them from following what they know to be the correct procedure and frequency. Are there environmental factors that prohibit them from doing it at the right frequency? Are there issues with the equipment they are using? Or are they simply not following the procedure they learned in the program?

NOTE

Robin had an interesting experience rolling out a project-management training program at a previous employer. People were given pre- and post-tests and showed a great deal of skill improvement. Robin wanted to see how they were applying those skills on the job and conducted a qualitative (anecdotal) survey. She asked one project manager how his leader liked the weekly reports recommended in the training program. He responded, "The first time I sent a report to my manager, he told me that he never wanted to see one of them again. So, I stopped sending them." We hope that this is not happening in clinical settings, but the example does allow you to see how environment and leaders can wreak havoc on the great training you have delivered!

Results

The final level, results, may be the only level in which senior-level leaders are interested. Although this is definitely important, Kirkpatrick (1996) warns against *only* evaluating this level, stating that as many levels as possible should be evaluated because each provides a different perspective into a training program. When evaluating results, you are looking for the final products of a training program. These could include, but are not limited to:

- Improved quality of care

- Reduction in costs

- Increased job satisfaction (and more importantly, reduced staff turnover)

- Any metrics/indicators the organization reports to external agencies (e.g., pressure ulcers or fall rates)

TABLE 6.1 Comparison of Kirkpatrick's Four Levels of Evaluation

	PROS	CONS
Reaction	Easy to measure Easy to make quick changes Assists in determining learner satisfaction and motivation	Does not provide an objective assessment of knowledge transfer
Learning	Relatively simple to create the instrument Quick and easy to gather data Provides an objective assessment of knowledge transfer	Does not ensure knowledge is transferred to on-the-job behavior
Behavior	Higher level of evaluation that assesses application/use of training concepts Potentially serves as an opportunity for the observer to correct behaviors in real time	Resource-consuming (time spent observing behavior) Does not ensure the program will have an impact on desired outcome (e.g., patient care or cost savings)
Results	Likely to be of greatest interest to senior-level leaders who manage the budget and other resources	Complex Resource-consuming (both time and money)

TABLE 6.2 Examples of Using Kirkpatrick's Four Levels of Evaluation

Scenario: Imagine you are given the task of assessing the effectiveness of an entire orientation program for new graduate nurses in an adult medical-surgical unit. The following questions are possible measurements that could be used to assess the various levels of evaluation.

Reaction	According to a Likert scale (e.g., on a scale of 1–5 [from Strongly Disagree to Strongly Agree]) survey, did the orientees like the orientation program? Based on anecdotal feedback from orientees, what could be changed about the orientation program to make it better?

Continues

TABLE 6.2 Examples of Using Kirkpatrick's Four Levels of Evaluation

Scenario: Imagine you are given the task of assessing the effectiveness of an entire orientation program for new graduate nurses in an adult medical-surgical unit. The following questions are possible measurements that could be used to assess the various levels of evaluation.

Learning	What was the measurable difference between pre-orientation and post-orientation tests used to assess cognitive knowledge in caring for adult patients with general medical and surgical problems?
	In a *simulated setting*, can nurses who have recently completed the orientation program perform the skills required in that unit?
Behavior	In the *actual unit*, can nurses who have recently completed the orientation program perform the skills required in that unit?
	What progress do preceptors, educators, and/or peers observe in the orientees with respect to clinical skills, decision-making, delegation, etc.?
Results	Did the reduction in orientation length yield the same degree of competency as nurses who completed a longer orientation?
	Do patients report a comparable degree of care received between nurses who recently completed orientation and those who have been working on the unit for an extended period of time?

You may note that many of the examples we used to describe Kirkpatrick's model involved assessing an orientation program rather than an individual's competency. Unfortunately, there is no single model that is widely accepted as the foundation of assessing a nurse's competency (that is, when they have successfully completed orientation). Some of the outcome measures of an orientation program's efficacy may involve nursing behaviors (for example, Kirkpatrick's learning and behavior levels can provide evaluation of an individual's performance). However, a holistic evaluation of an orientee is different from that of the organization, and the former is covered in Chapter 4.

Other Evaluation Models

Additional models (or methods) for evaluation include RSA, CIPP, ROI, and CBR. It may also be appropriate to choose a QI approach. (And you thought you had been in healthcare long enough to know all the abbreviations out there!) Let's briefly explore these.

RSA (Roberta S. Abruzzese)

The RSA model gets its name from the originator of the model, Roberta S. Abruzzese (1992). Her model is described in Table 6.3. It looks pretty similar to Kirkpatrick's model, right?

TABLE 6.3 RSA Model Overview

	DESCRIPTION	EXAMPLES
Process	Known as the "happiness index," this level measures learner satisfaction	Surveys Facilitated Group Discussions
Content	Measures the degree to which knowledge, skills, or attitudes were acquired or changed	Pre-Test/Post-Test Self-Assessments Simulations Case Studies
Outcome	Measures behavioral or performance change after returning to the clinical environment (typically assessed several months after the program)	Self-Assessments Direct Observation
Impact	Measures organizational results	Retention/Turnover Rates Quality Indicators Cost-Benefit Ratios
Total Program	Includes all other components (process, content, outcome, and impact) for a "big picture" view	Annual Reports

Source: Abruzzese (1992)

ROI (Return on Investment) and CBR (Cost-Benefit Ratio)

Determining an ROI or CBR allows you to place dollar signs into your evaluation data, which may speak with greater influence than other evaluation methods (depending on your audience). Both calculations provide similar data, but their formulas are slightly different:

ROI (%) = (Benefits − Costs) / Costs x 100

CBR = (Program Benefits) / (Program Costs)

The goal result in these calculations would be to obtain a number greater than or equal to 100% (for an ROI) or 1 (for a CBR). That would indicate the benefits (return) are greater than the costs (investments). Unfortunately, determining these values may be costly (pun intended). Consider the following two examples...

REAL-WORLD EXAMPLE: USING ROI/CBR IN YOUR EVALUATIONS, EASY EXAMPLE

Beth is a unit-based educator who would like to implement a preceptor training and development program because she believes it will enhance the orientation experience for both preceptors and orientees. She would like to provide a 4-hour class to 10 of her preceptors (who make $25/hour). Additionally, it will cost Beth about $500 in preparing content and developing learning materials. This means the cost of the program is $1,500 for both the preceptors' salaries along with the program development.

If she has a hunch that this could decrease the length of orientation (because the preceptors have gained additional skills), Beth could measure this impact in terms of salary. Let's say each preceptor oriented two nurses during the year, and these orientees had a shorter orientation than the previous year (by an average of two shifts, or 16 hours). If these orientees made $20/hour, that would mean they saved $6,400. Beth could display her results as follows:

$$ROI = (\$6{,}400 - \$1{,}500) / \$1{,}500 \times 100 = 327\%$$

$$CBR = \$6{,}400 / \$1{,}500 = 4.3$$

Either way, it is obvious the benefits (return) were well worth the costs (investment).

I call that an easy example because the number of factors to consider for calculation are few. Consider this example that falls on the other end of the spectrum...

REAL-WORLD EXAMPLE: USING ROI/CBR IN YOUR EVALUATIONS, DIFFICULT EXAMPLE

Dena is unit-based educator who is frustrated with the difficulty orientees experience in constructing complex intravenous line set ups in an intensive care unit. She would like to standardize the process among all of the units and create charts and figures the orientees could use as a reference (rather than learning and re-learning various approaches from different preceptors—a time-consuming endeavor).

To determine an ROI or CBR, Dena will need to consider, at minimum, the following factors in her calculations:

Cost/Investment—Dena's time (salary) spent in meetings with other units and stakeholders, chart/figure development, simulation supplies for teaching the new setup, etc.

Benefit/Return—Decreased time in training, decreased amount of wasted supplies, decreased cost of line infections (if any), etc.

Do you see the difficulty in collecting data in the latter example? Not only is there a large number of variables to measure, but assigning a dollar amount to some of the items (in this case, developing charts/figures or wasted supplies) can also be extremely challenging. Unfortunately, it may not be practical to use this type of evaluation for this particular project. Dena may have to settle for objective data only at the satisfaction level in this case.

QI (Quality Improvement)

QI has recently become a buzzword in many organizations as it allows clinicians who have relatively little experience in research to implement change projects rapidly, while ensuring valid statistical analysis of changes in outcome measures. Nursing professional development specialists could consider the use of these methods for evaluating the statistical significance of changes in metrics that are both objective and quantifiable in nature. There are several variations in methodological approaches (e.g., Six Sigma or Lean). Unfortunately, the process for engaging in rigorous QI projects is a bit more complex than we can place in one chapter. If you want more information on these methodologies, we invite you to contact your organization's quality improvement staff or check some of the reliable Internet sites we provide in the nearby sidebar.

KEY QI METHODS

The following are some of the key QI approaches you could choose to implement and where you can go to find more about them:

- *The Institute for Healthcare Improvement is a great resource dedicated to many facets of process and quality improvement within healthcare (http://www.ihi.org/)*

- *Six Sigma focuses on developing highly efficient, standardized processes (http://www.6sigma.us/)*

- *Lean is similar to Six Sigma but focuses more on reducing and eliminating waste (http://www.lean.org/)*

Summary of Models

It doesn't really matter which evaluation model or method you use as long as you use one that provides a systematic approach to evaluating program efficacy. They are all valid approaches, so you should pick one that makes sense to you, that you enjoy using, and that is practical given the resources you have at your disposal.

Additionally, you don't necessarily need to use every level of evaluation in every program. As you have hopefully seen in these examples, different levels are more appropriate in different situations, and some levels aren't even feasible in some cases. The goal is to have the greatest number of evaluation levels and/or the levels that demonstrate the greatest impact on patient care, but time and other resources will likely limit the degree to which this can be accomplished.

Evaluating an Organization's Orientation Program

Because we have already listed several examples of applying Kirkpatrick's model to an orientation program, let's now look at the big-picture, organizational view of evaluating an orientation program. As you know, hospitals, clinics, and other organizations come in various shapes and sizes with different infrastructures for a nursing professional development (or nursing education) department. Some organizations have adopted an entirely centralized department, some are completely decentralized, and some have eclectic combinations of the two. Smaller organizations may not even have a dedicated education department, but rather the nurse manager or director is responsible for staff development.

Regardless of the structure in your organization, the following methods and ideas can be modified to meet your needs. Also keep in mind that no one, single path should be considered the "right" way of doing orientation, and the most important consideration in evaluating an orientation program is answering the question: "Does the orientation program meet the needs of the organization while supporting its mission, vision, and values?"

Because we can't directly answer that important question for you, we want to provide you with additional questions that could help you answer that foundational one. Use Worksheet 6.1 to help you evaluate your organization's orientation program through a "define and discover" approach.

WORKSHEET 6.1 Evaluating an Organization's Orientation Program

DEFINE ("What is/are…")	DISCOVER ("How is your orientation program…")
…the organization's mission?	…contributing toward the organization achieving its mission?
…the organization's vision?	…helping the organization move toward its vision?
…the organization's values?	…assisting new employees in learning, incorporating, and supporting the values of the organization?
…the organization's greatest needs at this time (e.g., recent sentinel events, poor quality indicators, recommendations from an accrediting body survey, cost reduction, etc.)?	…addressing those needs?
…the principals (key stakeholders) in the organization, and what do they want out of the orientation program?	…meeting their goals and desires?
…other important factors to consider from your Assessment/Analysis performed in Chapter 2?	…meeting the needs identified in the Assessment/Analysis stage?
Final Question:	Final Question:
Are there any other components currently included in your orientation program that are not listed elsewhere?	If so, are they still needed, or should you consider removing them?

As you complete Worksheet 6.1, try to think of the outcome measures that will provide the highest level of objective evaluation while also being feasible. Doing this will help you stay on track to provide the principals (stakeholders) with evidence for changing or maintaining an orientation's activities. (It will also help you in preparing for a presentation or writing a publication when you discover a best practice worth sharing with others in the profession!)

Evaluating a Unit/Department's Orientation Program

Many of the concepts mentioned in evaluating an organization's orientation program also will be applicable to a unit/department's orientation program. However, the principals at this level may be different, so desired outcome measures may vary. For example, principals at the organizational level may include senior-level managers, while principals at the unit/departmental level may include preceptors and even patients.

Therefore, the "define and discover" approach used at this level will be very similar to the one used at the organizational level. However, we thought it was worth placing the worksheet here again with modifications already made to make it easier (and quicker!) to use—that's Worksheet 6.2.

WORKSHEET 6.2 Evaluating a Unit/Department's Orientation Program

DEFINE ("What is/are…")	DISCOVER ("How is your orientation program…")
…the unit/department's mission?	…contributing toward the unit/department achieving its mission?
…the unit/department's vision?	…helping the unit/department move toward its vision?
…the unit/department's values?	…assisting new employees in learning, incorporating, and supporting the values of the unit/department?
…the expected behaviors (i.e., competencies) of other staff in the unit/department?	…helping new hires learn those expectations and practice them consistently?
…the unit/department's greatest needs at this time (e.g., recent sentinel events, poor quality indicators, recommendations from an accrediting body survey, cost reduction, etc.)?	…addressing those needs?
…the principals (key stakeholders) in the unit/department, and what do they want out of the orientation program?	…meeting their goals/desires?
…other important factors to consider from your Assessment/Analysis as discussed in Chapter 2?	…meeting the needs identified in the Assessment/Analysis stage?

WORKSHEET 6.2 Evaluating a Unit/Department's Orientation Program

DEFINE ("What is/are…")	DISCOVER ("How is your orientation program…")
Final Question:	Final Question:
Are there any other components currently included in your orientation program that are not listed elsewhere?	If so, are they still needed, or should you consider removing them?

Evaluating an Individual's Orientation

Many evaluation strategies apply to an individual's orientation, too. The biggest difference will be that the behavior/outcome level (how they are performing in the clinical setting) is probably always being evaluated by a peer, preceptor, or educator and will determine *when* they are done with orientation (if you use a competency-based orientation program). This component is discussed more thoroughly in Chapter 4.

Additionally, unlike many programs in which evaluation is performed at the completion of the program, evaluating an individual's orientation experience will occur both during the process and at its completion.

You want to evaluate an individual's orientation experience for several reasons:

- Individuals may provide more insight into opportunities for improving an orientation program than aggregated survey data.

- Feedback can be acquired on preceptor performance.

- An individual's experiences during orientation will set the stage for his/her attitude toward his/her work environment, and you have the opportunity to check for any negative attitudes that may have surfaced.

- Evaluating an individual's experience (and making modifications, if required) demonstrates to the employee that you care about him/her as a person.

Following a similar format to the models discussed previously in this chapter, Table 6.4 is a guide to help evaluate an individual's orientation program and experience.

TABLE 6.4 Evaluating an Individual's Orientation

COMPONENT	EVALUATION ACTIVITIES
Satisfaction/Reaction/Process	Ask: How was your orientation experience? What did you like or dislike about it?
	Do: Post-Evaluation Survey with Likert scales as well as open-ended questions
Learning/Content	Ask: What was the best thing you learned in orientation? What were the easiest/hardest things to learn? What are your current strengths and areas for improvement?
	Do: Multiple-Choice Exam(s) assessing basic competencies, Acquire Preceptor Feedback
Behavior/Outcome	Ask: Do you see yourself performing patient care in a safe manner? What are your current strengths and areas for improvement?
	Do: Chart Audits, Direct Observation, Acquire Preceptor Feedback
Results/Impact	Not Applicable

*Note: These questions do not necessarily need to be asked in the past tense. You could (and should) modify these to ask them in present tense while the orientee is currently in orientation, too.

Tools/Handouts

Worksheet 6.3 can be used to help you evaluate your own program. It combines features of several models discussed in this chapter.

WORKSHEET 6.3 Questions to Guide Program Evaluation

COMPONENT	QUESTION TO ASK
Satisfaction/Reaction/Process	How will you measure learner satisfaction? *(surveys, Likert scales, open-ended responses, in-person or group interviews, immediately following program vs. delayed, etc.)*
Learning/Content	How will you measure the degree to which knowledge, skills, or attitudes were acquired or changed? *(pre-test and post-test exams, case studies, self-report, etc.)*

WORKSHEET 6.3 Questions to Guide Program Evaluation

COMPONENT	QUESTION TO ASK
Behavior/Outcome	How will you measure performance while in the clinical setting? *(direct observation, self-report, peer assessment, chart audits, etc.)*
Results/Impact	How will you measure the unit/organizational impact? *(cost [ROI/CBR], patient care [quality indicators or dashboards], etc.)*
Already Measuring	Are there any measures currently being assessed in the organization that could relate to your program? *(quality indicators, length of orientation, etc.)*
Who/When	Who is going to collect the data you would like measured, and when are they going to do it?
Other	What other components should be considered in evaluating this program?

Looking Beyond Orientation: A Note on Mentoring

Hopefully, this discussion on evaluating your orientation and onboarding programs has caused you to reflect a bit on the huge role your program plays in employees' success in the organization. This is a good time to begin thinking *beyond* the orientation experience and consider your role in the orientee's (and preceptor's!) transition out of those roles. Mentoring plays a significant role in this transition, and although an in-depth review of mentoring is beyond the scope of this book (and available from many other sources), we want to provide a few thoughts on the topic.

As a lead preceptor, Amy has a solid understanding of the difference between a preceptor and a mentor. "Just because a preceptor is a good teacher does not make them a good mentor and vice versa. Mentoring is more of a nurturing, emotionally comforting, mothering role than precepting is. Precepting is the building of knowledge and mentoring is the building of a support system."

"Mentoring is taking the relationship away from intense teacher to a concerned, interested, and nurturing coworker. Mentoring is interested in the coping, integrating, and building of new staff in their first year of employment. Mentoring allows for a more fluid conversation about how to tackle problems or navigate a unit's culture.

"For instance, my last mentee asked about the least costly way to utilize aspects of our health insurance. This isn't the common nursing knowledge that one would share when precepting but an important piece of information to that new employee seeking to make the best of their working environment."

Amy also encourages us to think back to when we started our careers with our current facility. By the 3-to 6-month mark, most employees are ready to dig deeper into what their employer has to offer in the way of climbing the ladder. They want to know: Who do you call to get your flu shot record? How does our yearly evaluation process work? Is there shared governance here? How does one navigate this medical insurance? Do the parking rules apply on weekends?

There is so much to a unit culture that is impossible to learn in just 6 to 12 short weeks. We know that information overload is not truly effective learning. Shoving information out into the room doesn't mean it is well absorbed to be utilized by new employees. There is a quote from Sydney J. Harris (an American journalist) about communication versus information that we would like to share with you. "The two words 'information' and 'communication' are often used interchangeably, but they signify quite different things. Information is giving out; communication is getting through."

Mentoring allows time for absorption. It allows the employee the time to get used to working for a facility and the typical care routines so they can start making connections, looking past the "how to do" and asking more in-depth questions.

Amy notes, "Mentoring is also about relating to both the needs of the mentor and the mentee. It takes away from the view of a teacher teaching 'at' you to a friend who has coffee 'with' you and with whom you can share your successes and concerns. The mentor and mentee relationship can actually be a wonderful two-way street. Mentors can take away just as much as the mentee can in personal or professional growth. Precepting is very one-sided in the learning and intensity within a defined set of time. Mentoring, if done in a way that addresses both needs of mentor and mentee, can last for an indefinite amount of time."

Amy and a search of best mentoring practices suggest that your mentor programs should consist of basic requirements such as goals for time together, mutual desire to build a relationship (for instance, both mentor and mentee should want to share with one another), and specified time limits for professional mentoring.

Basic requirements must be set to help the mentor know what your organization's goals are for mentoring. Basic requirements such as time frames, how often they should meet, and any monetary payment related to the mentor should be covered in an introductory session for potential mentors.

Goals for time together must have specific end dates. Beyond the goal of helping support nurses through their first year, mentees need focused attention to their goals for long-term professional development, and a senior nurse mentor can help with specific attainable goals.

We encourage you, as a staff educator (or other leader) involved in orientation, to think about the role you might play in helping build a mentoring program. Mentoring programs are natural extensions of orientation programs, and the mentor-protégé relationship could even start at the beginning of orientation!

Conclusion

Using a systematic evaluation approach, regardless of what specific model you use, will keep you on track and prevent overlooking an important component of the program. Structured evaluation, especially at higher and/or multiple levels, also demonstrates to others that you have a solid orientation program that wasn't created on a whim.

On a final note, in any organization, there will always be changes in leadership structure and/or new personnel in various decision-making positions. Keeping records of evaluation data will help in telling the story of how programs came to be what they are and prevent new people from "learning the hard way" when they want to try something new. Don't let all your hard work go to waste; keep records (at least summaries) of the evaluations you perform.

Questions for Reflection/Discussion

1. What processes do you currently have in place for evaluating your orientation program?

2. Do you feel your current orientation program meets the needs of your unit/department or organization?

3. Could you use additional models or levels of evaluation to more fully demonstrate the efficacy of your orientation program?

4. How do you see the use of multiple evaluation methods assisting you in building a case for additional orientation resources?

5. What processes do you currently have in place for evaluating an individual's orientation experience, and what (if anything) could be done to enhance this evaluation?

6. How would you describe the current mentoring environment? What improvements could be made to promote healthy mentor-protégé relationships?

KEY TAKEAWAYS

- *Evaluating an organization's, unit's, and individual's onboarding program/experience is vitally important in the continued efficacy of the onboarding process.*

- *Perform evaluations regularly and as close as possible to the end of a program.*

- *Seek feedback from multiple sources.*

- *Multiple models can be used to evaluate an onboarding program, and while each one has its strengths and weaknesses, using a variety of models and levels will likely be the best approach.*

- *Onboarding doesn't have to end once a new employee finishes his/her time with a preceptor—mentoring can be a key element to facilitate a successful transition to independent practice.*

References

Abruzzese, R. S. (1992). *Nursing staff development: Strategies for success.* St. Louis, MO: Mosby.

Kirkpatrick, D. (1996). Great ideas revisited: Revisiting Kirkpatrick's four-level model. *Training and Development, 50*(1), 54–59.

CHAPTER 7

Temporary Employees and Students

Introduction

Up to this point, we have been working under a major assumption that your orientees are being taught and onboarded as if they are permanent employees in your work area. Whether they are new graduates, experienced nurses, or transferring from another department in the organization, we have assumed they will remain with you for the foreseeable future. However, in many organizations, a number of other people temporarily enter the system and require varying levels of training, orientation, and/or onboarding to function in their intended roles. Because the amount of time they spend in an organization or particular department could vary from hours to months and the amount of previous experience could range from pre-licensure to experienced nurse, we thought a chapter dedicated to these learners' unique considerations would be helpful for readers.

We organized the chapter into the following three categories of learners:

- **Travelers**—Nurses who are primarily employed by an external agency and are contracted for a temporary time period

- **Float Staff**—Nurses employed by another unit/department who are working in a different location for a few hours or an entire shift

- **Students**—Pre-licensure students receiving a clinical experience as part of their academic curriculum

We'll collectively refer to this group as "temporary employees and students" to shorten the list, even if that doesn't capture the full uniqueness of the various roles. It's also worth noting that while the staff educator's responsibilities for most of these roles are fairly similar, the manager's responsibilities are not. Briefly, according to most regulatory bodies, the manager is ultimately responsible for ensuring the competency of his/her employees. Therefore, the manager will be very involved in the hiring of travelers but might have little oversight of students because they are not employed by the organization.

Travelers

Traveler...per-diem...temporary nurse...contract staff...agency nurse... locum tenens...there are many different names and references for those nurses whose primary employment is through an external agency that contracts with a healthcare organization to provide temporary nursing staff. We'll refer to them as *travelers* because that seems to be the more common term.

Selecting Travelers in Collaboration With Managers

When a unit/department considers hiring travelers to meet staffing needs, the staff educator and manager should work together to identify the preferred training and experience level of the potential travel nurses. You might consider bringing a competency assessment checklist or outline used for permanent staff orientation as a starting point and removing any skills that only permanent staff members would perform.

For example, if you work in a high acuity environment or one where you see patients with rare conditions, it might not be realistic to expect a traveler to have some of those experiences. You could remove these highly technical and/or rare skills from the expectations of your existing orientation document and then share that revised document with the manager. This revised document can serve as the minimum requirements needed that can be shared with the travel agency during the selection process. The staff educator might also be involved in the interview process, which typically occurs through phone- or web-based formats. The staff educator might bring a helpful perspective during the interview to help assess how he or she will fit with the unit.

Onboarding and Orientation Procedures

Once a travel nurse is selected and hired, the orientation period is typically very brief. At most, travelers tend to get 1 day of organization-wide orientation, and some of this can be done via web-based modules. Due to the brevity of this period, staff educators should be very intentional about communicating work logistics from the very first hour. For example, where should the traveler go on Day 1, and how will he/she access necessary systems and locations? In larger organizations, this responsibility might lie with the manager, centralized educators, and/or Human Resources specialists.

Following organization orientation, the unit or department onboarding is routinely conducted for two shifts with one of the permanent employees serving as a preceptor. During the unit-level onboarding period, travelers should be exposed to the types of patients they will be most likely to care for during their time in that unit. For example, if you work in a neuro unit that commonly cares for patients with seizures and continuous monitoring, the traveler should be exposed to at least one continuously monitored patient with seizures. An individual needs assessment completed by the traveler would be helpful for the preceptor and educator to identify beneficial patient care assignments during onboarding (and possibly to help the charge nurse identify appropriate patient assignments following onboarding). A partial example of an individual needs assessment is in Table 7.1. The educator populates the patient care knowledge and skills, and the traveler self-selects his/her experience level with each of the items.

TABLE 7.1 Individual Needs Assessment (Partial Example)

	KNOWLEDGE/SKILL	EXPERIENCE/FAMILIARITY 4 = Very Experienced 3 = Moderate Experience 2 = Minimal Exposure 1 = Never			
Neurological	Signs/symptoms and management of seizures	4	3	2	1
	Managing post-operative neurosurgical patients	4	3	2	1
	Anti-epileptic medications (e.g., levetiracetam, diazepam)	4	3	2	1
	...	...			
Pulmonary	Managing asthma and recognizing red-flag signs/symptoms	4	3	2	1
	Non-invasive positive airway pressures devices (e.g., BiPAP)	4	3	2	1
	Chest tubes	4	3	2	1
	...	...			
Vascular Access	Non-tunneled central venous catheters	4	3	2	1
	Peripherally inserted central catheters (PICC)	4	3	2	1
	Implantable ports	4	3	2	1
	...	...			

Staff educators can help the preceptors focus on teaching unit- and organization-specific knowledge as opposed to patient care activities. Travelers should be very familiar with providing patient care, so the focus of onboarding should be the unique items in that organization or unit. Examples include elements from Chapter 3 (Table 3.4) delineating items to cover on the first day and just-in-time resources (which are described in greater depth in the upcoming "Float Staff" section). You can think of travelers as similar to Experienced Eleanor (the experienced nurse) from Chapter 5.

Assessing and Ensuring Competency

Competency assessment of travelers is unique to each organization employing them, and it's largely up to you and management to determine how this step is conducted. Some travel agencies will have their employees take competency assessment exams (see sidebar). Additionally, many healthcare organizations will have travelers complete these assessments at the beginning of a travel assignment. Travel agencies might even provide resources to help their employees be successful on these exams.

COMPETENCY ASSESSMENT EXAMS FOR TRAVELERS

Although there is no one-size-fits-all competency assessment method, a few standardized exams for assessing competency are commonly used. These include:

- *Basic Knowledge Assessment Tool (BKAT)—Multiple-choice exam with versions for adult, pediatric, and neonatal critical care, adult progressive care, adult and pediatric emergency departments, and medical-surgical areas. Can be available for free in some situations at www.bkat-toth.org.*

- *AssessRx—Comprises several exams, including video-vignette based scenarios, previously known as the Performance Based Development System (PBDS). Developed by HealthStream; find more information at http://www.healthstream.com/solution/clinical-development/measure-validate-competency.*

- *Prophecy—Provides clinical, situational, and behavioral exams for dozens of settings and scenarios. More information can be found at http://info.prophecyhealth.com.*

Healthcare organizations can also develop hospital-specific assessments that could be completed at the centralized and/or unit levels (e.g., rhythm interpretation and medication administration tests). These latter assessments can be embedded into the previously described orientation and onboarding procedures.

All competency assessment documentation forms completed by the traveler (from medication administration tests at the unit level to intravenous medication pump skills check-offs at general orientation) should be stored by the hiring unit. Although the *quantity* of orientation-related documents you have for a traveler likely won't be as large as experienced nurses join your permanent staff, the *quality* should mimic that of experienced nurses. In other words, the types of documents you keep will be similar, but given travelers' limited orientation time, they won't complete as many assessments. Chapter 8 ("Regulatory Considerations") contains additional information on the storage of orientation-related documents.

NOTE

> *Because travelers are not full-time hires of the organization, it is important that they not attend regular staff meetings. By having them attend these meetings, you would be treating them as full-time employees, and that can cause co-employment issues for your organization. If you have a traveler and are not sure what meetings the person can or cannot attend, contact your Human Resources department. They will be able to provide guidance for you on the expectations.*

Even though travelers are not required to attend staff meetings, if new practices, procedures, and/or equipment are introduced into the work area, they *will* need to have their competency assessed on these changes. Anyone who is providing patient care within an organization must be deemed competent to provide that care. Unfortunately, the rigor of competency-assessment methods and corresponding documentation moves us into a gray area. As a couple of examples, imagine your unit switched manufacturers of intravenous (IV) catheters and purchased a new style. Chances are high that an experienced traveler has been exposed to different styles of IV catheters and might not need to attend an inservice with the permanent staff (although they should be invited and welcomed to attend). Alternatively, let's say the organization's cardiothoracic surgeons have recently made major changes to the post-operative standards of care for cardiac patients. If the traveler completed orientation before the changes took place and currently provides care for these patients, he/she would need to be included in any training provided to the permanent staff. Documentation of the traveler's competency assessment for these changes can remain with the rest of your documents for this learning activity.

Float Staff

Primarily in hospitals, as opposed to clinics or long-term care facilities, float staff are employees of one unit/department who spend anywhere from a few hours to a whole shift in a different department that is under-staffed. A house supervisor typically oversees the needs of the hospital and identifies which units could "float" a few nurses to another unit to ensure a more balanced patient:nurse ratio and enhance patient safety and quality.

There are also some organizations that have a "float pool" composed of nurses employed by the organization but not a specific patient care unit. Some of these employees might work on a different unit every day while others might spend several weeks or months on one unit filling in for nurses who are temporarily out on leave (e.g., maternity leave). You might think of float pool nurses as a middle ground between travelers and employees who float only as needed in rare situations. If you're a staff educator working in a float pool department, the ADDIE model described in previous chapters will be very applicable to your orientation programs; however, you'll also want to build strong working relationships with staff educators in the other departments in order to optimize the onboarding experience of your nurses.

For most nurses, floating to another unit is extremely undesirable. Floating to another unit tends to occur when the receiving unit is short-staffed, meaning the patient:nurse ratio is likely higher than usual. This increased workload places additional pressures not only on the floated nurse but also on the nurses on the unit to whom the floated nurse must reach out for assistance in identifying resources, locating supplies, and understanding population-specific patient needs. Although nurses are great critical thinkers with well-developed skills for adaptability, attempting to do one's work in a new environment is very challenging for anyone. Many of the subconscious actions that become routine (i.e., second nature) to us are thrown out the proverbial window, and the accompanying increases in cognitive workload are enormous.

But even with all these challenges, floating will remain a necessity of our healthcare system due to unpredictable fluctuations in patient acuity, patient census, and staffing. So, what can the staff educator do to help alleviate some of these challenges? Staff educators can help by:

- Managing the culture
- Creating just-in-time resources
- Facilitating cross-training

Managing the Culture

Managing the culture is perhaps the most challenging aspect of improving the floating experience. Along with the nurse managers and other unit leadership, the staff educator can help direct-care clinicians to appreciate the macro-system of the healthcare environment, as well as teach and role model helpful interpersonal communication strategies. For the former, consider some of the "Different Perspectives on Floating" (see sidebar), especially for employees who are internally motivated.

DIFFERENT PERSPECTIVES ON FLOATING

As leaders, staff educators should try to promote a more positive culture of floating by reminding staff of the following:

- *It's an opportunity to be exposed to a new patient population.*

- *Staff will meet new colleagues and expand their professional network.*

- *Nurses can help out their fellow nurses in the organization.*

- *Ask the manager or higher leadership to thank (in person) the floated staff for being willing to help another unit.*

Regarding the teaching and role modeling of beneficial communication strategies, staff educators can work with nurses in the department to focus on: (a) being very intentional when a floated staff member comes to your unit and (b) expressing the need for assistance with an unfamiliar environment or task. As far as being intentional with a floated staff member, some organizations have set up a "buddy" system whereby the charge nurse on the receiving unit assigns one of the unit's nurses to be the point person for the floated nurse. Both the floated nurse and buddy nurse are aware of this designation, and the buddy nurse can be intentional about frequently checking on the floated nurse. The "Is This Dose Too Big?" sidebar provides an example of how this can work.

In the opposite situation, when a nurse floats to different unit, he/she should be intentional about receiving the necessary assistance to safely provide patient care. Staff educators can work with orientees and existing staff members to feel comfortable asking for help. The "How Do You Feed a Baby?" sidebar provides an example of how this can work.

IS THIS DOSE TOO BIG?

I (Alvin) remember a time when a neonatal ICU nurse floated to the pediatric ICU. Even though the charge nurses typically tried to provide a patient assignment with infants to floated neonatal ICU nurses, it didn't work out that day. The neonatal ICU nurse had an adolescent patient, who was a very stable patient but just much larger than the floated nurse's usual patient.

I had introduced myself, thanked her for being willing to float to our unit, and offered to help with anything she might need. I jokingly said, "Sorry you have such a large patient! Let me know if you want to run anything by me." She smiled and said, "You're going to think I'm an idiot, but did I draw up the right amount of acetaminophen (Tylenol)? This dose just looks too big!" We both laughed, and I confirmed the dose was correct.

This was a great reminder that even simple tasks can seem very complicated when performing them in a new environment. Some scripted phrases that could be beneficial include:

- *"Thank you so much for helping us out today! Please let me know if you need anything."*
- *"What questions do you have that I could help with?"*
- *"How are you feeling about your assignment?"*
- *"Can I get any supplies for you or help with documentation?"*

HOW DO YOU FEED A BABY?

I (Alvin) remember a time when I was floated to the neonatal ICU. As a pediatric ICU nurse, I have been floated there many times in my career, and we also see lots of infants in the pediatric ICU. Even though I thought I had a pretty good grasp on what I'd be doing that day, I made sure I introduced myself to the nurses working near me and made a comment along the lines of, "If it looks like I'm doing anything out of the ordinary, please feel free to let me know."

I was performing one of the routine feedings (which most babies have every 3 hours), and one of the neonatal ICU nurses was looking over at me and asked, "Have you ever fed a newborn before?" (Being a pediatric nurse for 10 years, certified in pediatric critical care, and almost done with my PhD, my first thought was, "Are you kidding me?!?! Of course, I have!!" But then I remembered I did say they could give me feedback.) So, I responded with, "Yes, but do you have suggestions on how I could improve?" She proceeded to provide me with some new techniques that I had not used previously, which made her feel more comfortable with my handling of "their" babies and reminded me that there's always something new to learn in this profession!

Creating Just-in-Time Resources

A common practice to assist nurses floated to a new unit is to have a physical or electronic just-in-time resource document available. These documents provide concise but essential information to help float staff provide high-quality patient care. Check out Worksheet 7.1 to help you identify several important elements we recommend for a just-in-time resource. We recommend creating the resources with input from nurses in your department and staff educators from other departments (this could even be a good activity for an organization-wide staff educator meeting).

WORKSHEET 7.1
Guide to Creating Just-in-Time Resources for Float Staff

	RESPONSE
People	*Who are the most frequently contacted people, and how can they be reached?*
	Consider starting with charge nurses, physicians, pharmacy, and housekeeping.
Routines	*What specific routines exist on the unit?*
	Consider whether there are "standard" times for activities like medication administration, vital sign measurement, and laboratory specimen collection.
Supplies	*What is the location of commonly used supplies?*
	Consider adding the location of the most commonly used supplies, such as IV supplies, linens, or the nutrition room, and provide any passcodes for doors that are locked.
Policies & Procedures	*Are there any policies or procedures that are different from the rest of the organization?*
	Consider unique documentation practices in addition to patient care procedures.
Patients	*Are there patient-population-specific signs and symptoms of which to be aware?*
	Consider whether there are some red flags that could pose serious harm to patients if not recognized and managed.

ADDITIONAL FLOATING RESOURCES

If you're looking for some examples of what others have created for their floating needs, you can check out the following references:

- *Bates, K. J. (2013). Floating as a reality: Helping nursing staff keep their heads above water.* MedSurg Nursing, 22*(3), 197.*

- *Cita, B. (2010). Top ten tips for fearless floating.* Nursing2016, 40*(2), 57–58.*

- *Crowell-Grimme, T., & Garner, L. A. (2007). Creating a guide for float nurses.* Nursing2016, 37*(12), 17.*

- *Good, E., & Bishop, P. (2011). Willing to walk: A creative strategy to minimize stress related to floating.* Journal of Nursing Administration, 41*(5), 231–234.*

- *Roach, J. A., Tremblay, L. M., & Carter, J. (2011). Hope floats: An orthopaedic tip sheet for float pool nurses.* Orthopaedic Nursing, 30*(3), 208–212.*

Facilitating Cross-Training

Closely related to the concept of floating is the idea of cross-training. While floating is a temporary solution associated with many negative emotions, cross-training is intentional, planned, and some employees typically *want* to do it. Cross-training involves formally orienting and onboarding an employee to a work area that is not the employee's primary work area. For example, it is not uncommon for a medical ICU nurse to be cross-trained to the surgical ICU. In this case, the nurse is primarily employed by the medical ICU and works the majority of his/her time there. When the surgical ICU is short-staffed, the cross-trained employee would be the first person to float to that unit. In some organizations, there are strong relationships between units where, in order to maintain a high degree of competency in multiple units, a nurse in Unit A will work two of the three weekly shifts in Unit A and spend the other shift in Unit B. Unit B performs the same activity in reverse with one of its nurses spending two shifts in Unit B and one shift in Unit A.

Cross-training can overcome the barrier of increased cognitive workload associated with floating to an unknown environment because a formal orientation (even if very brief) has been planned. Therefore, employees can find the resources and supplies needed to do their job. Additionally, they tend to become more familiar with the nurses working in the other unit and feel more comfortable reaching out to them for assistance.

Depending on your organization's needs, facilitating cross-training experiences could be as complex as designating a cohort of employees who receive extended onboarding in another unit (or several units). It could also be as simple as scheduling a new employee for a couple shifts (or a couple weeks) during orientation/onboarding to train on another unit. For example, if a new employee is hired by a newborn nursery in an organization where those nurses are intermittently floated to the post-partum floor and neonatal ICU, it might make sense for the new employee to spend several shifts during orientation with a preceptor in those other two units.

Given the brevity and intentionality of these learning opportunities, we have created Worksheet 7.2 for determining how to organize the onboarding experiences for these situations. We also recommend referring back to Worksheet 7.1 regarding just-in-time resources for float staff to aid educators and preceptors as to where to focus onboarding activities.

WORKSHEET 7.2
Organizing a Cross-Training Onboarding Program

	RESPONSE
High-Priority Work Areas	*Which units/departments in the organization have similar patient populations? Which units/departments frequently require float staff?*
	Consider organizing a formal cross-training program between similar units, as well as with those units that frequently require float staff.
Personal Preferences	*Are there employees on the unit who are interested in cross-training on another unit?*
	Some nurses might be interested in expanding their clinical skills or learning more about additional populations. (For example, pediatric ICU nurses working in a medical-surgical setting might want to cross-train to the cardiac ICU in preparation for their CCRN certification exam.) Consider cross-training these nurses first.
Timing	*When would cross-training best be provided?*
	Think about whether new employees should receive cross-training to another unit while in their initial onboarding period because their time is "protected" for this period. Also consider orientee influx in the other unit/department and whether cross-training should occur at a time of the year when the unit's preceptors are not as busy.

WORKSHEET 7.2
Organizing a Cross-Training Onboarding Program

	RESPONSE
Patients, Policies, and Procedures	*What are the top 5 (or 10) most common diagnoses and/or treatments seen in your unit/department?*
	Ensure these diagnoses, treatments, and any relevant policies/procedures are covered in the learning activities, whether via precepted patient care during onboarding or through didactic materials, such as a class or an online module.
Competency Assessment	*How will you assess the cross-trained employee's competence?*
	Although floating for a single shift doesn't tend to involve a formal competency assessment, the pre-planned format of cross-training programs permits some degree of competency assessment (e.g., a knowledge and skills checklist for a preceptor, cross-trained employee's attendance at the unit's skills fair, or regularly working shifts in the other unit).

Students

Even though having clinical nursing students on one's unit can be challenging, this can actually be a great recruitment strategy for the unit while also ensuring a steady pipeline of future nurses. Staff educators can alleviate some of challenges by implementing procedures that disrupt routine care as little as possible. These procedures include activities like collaborating with the academic affiliates on long-term plans for accommodating students, preparing staff for differences in clinical instructor versus preceptor approaches to teaching, and ensuring that staff members are aware of each state's scope of practice related to non-licensed personnel.

Collaborating With Academic Affiliates

There are two primary collaboration activities between healthcare organizations and the academic affiliates who send their students there for training: (1) centralized discussions of "big picture" items and coordination of contracts, and (2) unit-level coordination of daily/weekly/monthly activities for students and their educators.

Centralized work begins with discussions of determining from which schools the organization will accept students. Decisions might be made based on proximity, number of students who need experiences throughout the year, perceived quality of the program, pass rate trends on the national licensure exam, and type of program (i.e., associate degree, baccalaureate degree, etc.), among others. Centralized staff educators can contribute to these conversations with knowledge of each unit's capacity for students. For example, you might know that the orthopedic unit added several new beds and will be hiring many new nurses in the next 6 months to meet the increased patient census—this unit probably isn't an ideal learning situation for students at this time.

Once the organization has identified the schools with which it will participate, a legal contract will be signed by both parties. This contract will contain items such as licensure and orientation of academic clinical instructors, liability insurance, governing law and venue, indemnification, and students' immunization status. A few schools and clinical sites have made their contracts and policies available online. Try searching for something similar to "clinical affiliation nursing schools agreement."

Dedicated education units (DEUs) are becoming increasingly popular because they help alleviate the nursing faculty shortage in the United States. Within DEUs, permanent staff members regularly serve as clinical instructors for students. This steady stream of students helps create a culture of teaching, and there tends to be a greater emphasis on purposefully preparing staff to be excellent teachers. Similarly, some organizations have full-time employees who serve as clinical instructors in multiple units (typically, their salaries are reimbursed by the academic affiliate). A benefit of this approach is that permanent unit staff recognize the clinical instructor as "one of their own" (in contrast to academic clinical instructors whom staff nurses might see only infrequently) and tend to have improved communication. In both of these situations, staff educators should build strong working relationships with those working and/or supervising on the units, because the staff educator helps ensure all preceptors are competent to provide high-quality care and teach students to do the same.

Further, there are many items that RNs are competent to do during work hours that are very different when they enter the clinical instructor role. For example, if an employee has been deemed competent to operate a point-of-care glucometer, when that same person is working in the role of a clinical instructor, that person might have to reestablish competency with the glucometer in this new role. As an educator, you might need to consider whether the time to reevaluate the instructor's competency is worth the clinical time saved in having the instructor (as opposed to employee) sign off for the student. Some organizations even provide different electronic health record identifiers for nurses serving as both an employee and as a clinical instructor.

Whether or not you work in a DEU, the staff educator's responsibilities for unit-level coordination might involve:

- Determining appropriateness of having students

- Identifying appropriate days/shifts to welcome students

- Helping preceptors identify patient assignments that yield optimal learning opportunities

- Discussing current academic status (e.g., first-semester students versus final-semester students) with charge nurses and bedside staff to establish scope of practice

Clinical Instructor Supervision vs. Preceptor Models

Students may enter a unit/department in a couple of ways: as a group under the direction of an academic clinical instructor, or individually under the direction of an employed nurse serving as a preceptor. In both cases, the primary direct care nurse (and possibly the charge nurse) should be apprised of the student's previous experiences and goals for the day. Knowing this will help the unit's staff provide learning opportunities of greatest benefit to the students.

In the clinical-instructor-supervision scenario, ideally, the clinical instructor carries the responsibility of seeking out ideal learning opportunities for students. The staff educator (and/or charge nurse) can assist the clinical instructor with this by touching base at the beginning of the shift and intermittently throughout the shift to discuss items such as: a) whether non-routine activities are planned (e.g., bedside procedures), b) the presence of patients with interesting diagnoses or clinical findings, and c) organizational resources that would be beneficial to students' learning (e.g., instructional videos or learning activity materials for current staff).

Under the preceptor model for nursing students, one of the organization's permanent employees serves as a preceptor for the student. The student might be spending a single shift or an entire semester with the preceptor (the latter being more common in the final semester of a nursing program). The staff educator can facilitate optimal learning experiences here by preparing the preceptor for the unique task of teaching students. As opposed to precepting a new graduate nurse who is a licensed clinician working toward independent practice, students require a higher level of supervision throughout their learning experience. Because students are not licensed individuals, most nurses do not permit students to perform as much independent work as a new graduate nurse. (For additional directions on scope of practice, we suggest you check with your organization's policies on students and trainees.) To ensure a great learning opportunity, the preceptor should consider the strategies listed in "Tips for Precepting Student Nurses."

PRECEPTOR POINTER:
TIPS FOR PRECEPTING STUDENT NURSES

Due to the limited scope of practice of non-licensed personnel, preceptors can engage in the following behaviors to optimize the learning experience of students:

- *Let them know that this isn't a test—Since you're asking them questions, make sure they know that it is OK to give an incorrect answer. Your concerns are a) doing the right thing for the patient and b) helping the student increase his/her knowledge and skills.*

- *Talk while tasking—Verbalize your thoughts regarding current activities, upcoming activities, and task rationales. This will help students to begin "thinking like a nurse" and is colloquially referred to as "making the invisible visible."*

- *Ask "Why ?"—Posing multiple questions to students helps them link their didactic training with the practice arena. A major challenge for students is the gap that seems to exist between the classroom and clinical environment. By asking questions (without the expectation that the student be right), the preceptor can identify and correct any misconceptions and promote critical thinking.*

- *Look for unique opportunities—Preceptors can connect students with nearby colleagues who might be caring for patients different from the preceptor's assignment. Preceptors can also look for opportunities for students to visit other departments (e.g., following a patient to radiology or the operating room).*

- *Promote interprofessional activities—Consider how students can be included in interprofessional rounding, discussions, and participation.*

- *Provide feedback—Just as licensed orientees want feedback on their performance, so do students. We recommend the feedback be as encouraging as possible. We all remember how challenging nursing school was, and hearing "I think you'll make a great nurse" from a staff member can really help with the endurance needed to finish school.*

- *Allow for time for processing—Because students haven't typically been exposed to the variety and frequency of emotionally taxing situations with which nurses deal, students need time to share their experiences with someone who can listen, provide reassurance, and validate the interventions, tasks, thoughts, and emotions that are executed rapidly (and seemingly too rapidly for a student). Some people refer to this as "reflection," and if you're interested in learning more, you might check out Gwen Sherwood and Sara Horton-Deutsch's book* Reflective Practice: Transforming Education and Improving Outcomes *(2012).*

- *Establish boundaries—Preceptors should explicitly communicate their expectations of each student's roles, tasks, and level of independence. Preceptors are serving as role models, educators, socializers, and protectors, and explicit communication helps sustain this large amount of multi-tasking. Check out the upcoming "Scope of Practice Considerations" section for additional details.*

PRECEPTOR POINTER:
MAINTAINING YOUR (AND THE STUDENT'S) SANITY

It's easy for preceptors to grow increasingly frustrated with student nurses because they have to be reminded of each individual step in a task. We expect students to memorize the "how to set up a sterile field" in school in a step-by-step learning style, but applying those steps in a complex environment and with new equipment can be extremely challenging. A great way to maintain your sanity (and that of the student) is to focus on completing *tasks one step at a time.*

When you put the instructions in language they are accustomed to hearing, it helps the student be more successful. If you spit out the instructions all at once, the student gets frustrated because he/she has no reference for it. Taking each task one step at a time helps them remember it in the future or at least have an instinct that they have seen this before. Consider the following exemplar for how to communicate with the student about an intravenous (IV) medication administration scenario:

"When I am concerned about adding new continuous IV medications to the patient's continuous drips, I look in our intranet formulary, click on this icon [demonstrating the location on the computer], hover over that toolbar, and click 'IV Compatibilities.' Now I add each IV medication, and once that is completed, I hit the red compile button because I like seeing compatibility that way."

Just as floating is associated with many negative attitudes, many permanent staff members perceive having students on the unit as a negative experience. These negative attitudes, which are easily recognized by the students, can impede the students' learning experience. Don't get us wrong...we understand what it's like to be over-worked and under-resourced, and then to have students on the unit who need time from us that we just can't seem to find! We wish we could provide your staff with some free time as a thank you for buying this book (we tried to negotiate sending you a traveler for a few days to give your preceptors a break, but our publisher said it was too expensive). But we do have a few thoughts to share on the perspectives we try to remember when having students with us (especially when they are unexpected guests):

- I was a student once, and I needed good preceptors just as much as these students do now.

- If I don't teach them how to do it, who will?

- What if this student is *my* nurse one day? I want to ensure we have an intelligent cadre of nurses in the future.

- It's OK to ask, "That's a good question—let me complete this first, then let's discuss your question." Students know we're busy, and this question shows we respect the student while prioritizing patient (or self!) care.

We know these questions and thoughts won't resolve all the problems in our resource-constrained environments. But especially for those who are intrinsically motivated, this can be a starting point for some beneficial reflection.

Scope of Practice Considerations

Each state has its own nurse practice act that guides the scope of practice for licensed nurses in that state. Some of this might also pertain to student issues. For example, Ohio's nurse practice act requires at least 2 years of experience for registered nurse preceptors who are teaching nursing students (Ohio Administrative Code Chapter 4723-5, Nursing Education Programs). Other state health boards can also have laws mandating scope of practice; for example, students might not be allowed independent access to automated medication dispensing systems (e.g., Pyxis™) due to Board of Pharmacy rules. To find what's allowed in your state, we recommend opening your state's practice acts from Nursing, Pharmacy, and Medicine, then searching for words like "student" and "preceptor." Organizations can set stricter standards than the state; however, they cannot permit more than the state allows.

When students are exposed to multiple preceptors, it can be easy for student nurses to push the limits of their scope because the preceptors might not recognize all the nuances of students' scope of practice. Roles and tasks might vary on a given shift (or for higher acuity patients). For example, if a student nurse is asked to flush a peripheral intravenous catheter, the student might agree because the task seems simple and he/she could complete it independently. However, performing the task without direct oversight from a licensed, qualified preceptor is technically outside the student's scope of practice. Establishing boundaries at the beginning of a shift and communicating frequently will help avoid these inappropriate situations.

From a documentation perspective, unit-based educators do not need to keep competency records for students who are taught by the academic affiliate instructor. In contrast, if you're working on a unit where students are primarily taught by a permanent staff member, remain in the unit for a prolonged period (e.g., several months during the student's final semester of school), and are permitted to do a broader range of skills, it's probably safer to keep competency assessment records for these students.

Conclusion

In addition to having a complex nursing environment in which to operate, we sometimes find ourselves working with others who are not the "regular" crew. To that end, it is important that we are prepared to receive travelers, floaters, and students into our crew for a shift or a series of shifts. Understanding the unique circumstances of each type of new crew member helps us help them and helps us all take great care of our patients.

Keep focused on the competencies required and expectations set for a regular crew member, and help your new crew understand and demonstrate those competencies and expectations.

Questions for Reflection/Discussion

1. What types of temporary employees and students frequent your organization or unit/department?

2. What procedures and resources are in place (and what could be added) to ensure the success of temporary employees and students?

3 How strong are the interdepartmental relationships among the locations that give and receive float staff?

4. What might a formal cross-training program look like in your organization?

5. What are the attitudes and experiences of permanent staff regarding the onboarding of temporary employees and students?

6. Does your state and/or organization have specific guidelines limiting the scope of practice for students (or the qualifications of their preceptors)?

KEY TAKEAWAYS

- *Make a game plan with your managers to understand what the goal is for each temporary staff member's employment and how much time will be allotted for successful onboarding.*

- *Be sure to give support to temporary staff members during their time in your clinical area. (Evaluating temporary staff can be even easier if core staff members understand the goals of their time on the unit.)*

- *Even though standardizing a competency list is helpful, don't forget the past experience of the temporary staff, as it can change the game plan of the preceptor's priorities.*

- *Consider how you can best use orientation time to help the temporary staff be most successful in your clinical area. If the temporary staff member is going to have 8 hours of orientation, a clear plan needs to be in place to help them be successfully safe after that time. Keep it simple and standardized so you will know what is working and what needs more work.*

References

Ohio Administrative Code. Chapter 4723-5, Nursing Education Programs. Last revised 12/19/2016.

Sherwood, G. D., & Horton-Deutsch, S. (2012). *Reflective practice: Transforming education and improving outcomes.* Indianapolis, IN: Sigma Theta Tau International.

CHAPTER 8

Regulatory Considerations

Introduction

If you've been in nursing for even a short period of time, you're very aware of the plethora of rules, regulations, governing boards, accrediting bodies, etc., that set practice standards for what you do as a nurse. From basic scope-of-practice standards such as delegation to the more complex requirements such as annual competency assessments, external entities play a huge role in ensuring safe patient care. Many nurses (and especially nurse managers) get antsy at the thought of a visit from a regulatory body, and there is likely a lot of tension throughout the organization during a review. It can be easy to think of these agencies trying to scrutinize every little detail to the point of being just plain ridiculous.

We want to start this discussion on regulatory issues by changing the perspective just a little. Rather than looking at a regulatory body's purpose as attempting to make your life as difficult as possible, try to see them through a patient's eyes. The regulatory bodies are simply trying to protect patients and their loved ones from poor healthcare practices. And guess what? If you follow the tips we've outlined in this chapter, you'll already have your ducks in a row, and there will be no need to worry about issues during a visit from these agencies.

To help with this, start by recognizing that most regulatory agencies do not tell you *how* to do something but rather *what* you need to do. Take the example of The Joint Commission's requirement for staff training related to caring for patients of different ages. Most nurses are probably aware of this requirement, and many organizations provide a unique, annual age-specific education module to all direct-care providers. However, in looking at The Joint Commission's requirement (at least as it was displayed at the time this book was written), it states that education should be specific to the populations served by the organizations. This could imply that not only should different age groups be included but perhaps also different cultures (which we now know they do include based on subsequent recommendations from The Joint Commission). The other problem with this distinct education module is that the guideline does not require a separate piece of education. You could consider incorporating age- and culture-specific information into educational initiatives already occurring (e.g., educating on different sizes of restraints, or building case studies that involve patients of different cultures).

The point we're trying to make is that you shouldn't build mountains that you can't climb, so try to integrate as many accrediting-body and regulatory requirements as possible into fewer diverse education modules rather than having a separate module for each standard. Table 8.1 has a quick example of what we mean by combining these modules. The bottom line is that you will find overlapping regulations, requirements, etc., so build them into existing modules where the content makes sense. This will make you and your staff members a lot happier.

In this chapter, we'll cover key concepts related to accrediting bodies, state and federal government mandates, and finally documentation. There will definitely be some overlap in these areas, but Figure 8.1 describes what makes these distinct.

TABLE 8.1
Two Examples of Combining Multiple Regulatory Requirements Into One Education Module

MODULE AND CONTENT	CONTENT MANDATED BY	RATIONALE
Safety Curriculum: Employee safety behaviors (e.g., wearing personal protective equipment, cleaning up hazardous materials) Patient safety goals (e.g., patient identification, healthcare acquired infections)	Occupational Safety and Health Administration (OSHA) The Joint Commission (TJC)	Because both of these organizations have expected safety behaviors and goals, you could combine these (and even organizations!) into one module discussing "safety" rather than having two separate modules.
Restraints Across the Lifespan: Indications, application, and monitoring of restraints for patients of all age groups.	The Joint Commission (TJC) Centers for Medicare & Medicaid Services (CMS)	TJC requires both restraint and population-specific training while CMS requires restraint training.

NOTE

Disclaimer: We are not licensed attorneys. In fact, we are not attorneys at all, nor do we play attorneys on television! We are not providing any type of legal or regulatory advice. If you have questions about a certain situation, please contact your nursing leader and/or Human Resources.

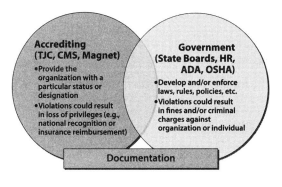

FIGURE 8.1

*Distinctions between accrediting and governmental bodies.
(Note that documentation's role is to provide evidence to demonstrate compliance with regulatory standards.)*

Accreditation Standards

Accrediting bodies are those external organizations that provide a particular credential, certification, or status for an organization based upon the fulfillment of a minimum set of criteria. Different organizations (and even departments) have different accrediting bodies that could set these expectations. For example, the American Nurses Credentialing Center (ANCC) can designate an entire hospital system as achieving Magnet® status, while the American Association of Critical-Care Nurses (AACN) could designate an intensive care unit as achieving the Beacon Award for Excellence. The intensive care unit receiving the Beacon award that exists within a hospital system holding a Magnet designation would be responsible for meeting expectations set by both accrediting bodies.

While some of these accrediting bodies are responsible for recognizing excellence (such as the aforementioned Magnet and Beacon recognitions), other accrediting bodies provide certain privileges (e.g., the Centers for Medicare and Medicaid Services [CMS] sets expectations of organizations that wish to receive insurance reimbursement). In contrast to the governmental (legal) issues that follow this section, an organization's participation in the accrediting process is typically voluntary, albeit highly desired. They all contain a wide variety of requirements, but we want to briefly focus on the expectations they set for newly hired employees.

We do not wish to provide an exhaustive list of expectations from each of these organizations for two reasons:

1. The organizations can change their expectations at any time, so it is best for you to find the most current guidelines.

2. Each organization may interpret the guidelines slightly differently.

Most organizations make their accrediting manuals available to employees. If you don't know where to find a particular manual, contact your manager or compliance officer for additional information. Once you find the source manual, search through it looking for words like *orientation*, *training*, *initial*, *competency*, and *hire*. As you find these, write those statements down and begin building a list of things that must be included. Once you extract these statements from all the agencies to which you report, you will have all the necessary guidelines to ensure you can withstand an audit (as long as you also implement their requests and document performance of them). Although this might sound like a lot, you'll probably quickly find that many of the external agencies have quite a bit of overlap (such as waived testing or restraint requirements).

The Joint Commission

If you work in a hospital, home care, or behavioral health, you are well aware of The Joint Commission (TJC) and its many requirements. Because this likely will apply to the majority of readers, we will use this accrediting body as an example. However, many other accrediting bodies are specific to smaller organizations, such as college health clinics and ambulatory surgery centers (Accreditation Association for Ambulatory Health Care), community health centers (Community Health Accreditation Program), and so on. Accreditation by these organizations designates your facility as an organization where patients can expect to receive high-quality care. Because of this, many organizations focus on active improvement work (in addition to meeting basic requirements) to continue pushing the envelope on what is considered quality care.

Regarding orientation, TJC outlines several requirements as being necessary. One of the most basic requirements is simply that the organization provides an orientation to staff. TJC offers a few specifics of what must be included in that orientation, but there is also a lot of freedom in what can be included. Typically, their guidelines ask that you train new personnel in the following specific areas and document successful completion of the training (TJC, 2017):

- Basic job duties
- Pain management
- Cultural diversity
- Patient rights and ethical issues
- Performing waived tests
- Restraints

Centers for Medicare & Medicaid Services

Similar to TJC, the Centers for Medicare & Medicaid Services (CMS) sets minimum expectations; however, CMS does not require the degree of improvement work that TJC does. Instead, CMS sets Conditions of Participation (CoP), which are minimum requirements that must be met to receive reimbursement for patients using Medicare or Medicaid. If these CoPs are not met, the organization risks losing its major funding source, as other insurance companies will also cease reimbursement activities to follow suit with CMS.

With respect to orientation, CMS requires documentation of the following non-exhaustive items (CMS, 2015):

- Initial training and competency assessment
- Abuse and neglect
- Blood and blood product administration
- Medication preparation and administration
- Restraints and seclusion

In addition to basic requirements for various organizations (e.g., hospitals have specific criteria), some programs within organizations have additional requirements (e.g., if hospitals manage patients receiving solid organ transplants, transplant-specific criteria will also be required of the hospital).

Other Regulatory Bodies

In addition to these major accrediting bodies, other agencies may also regulate activities at your organization. For example, the American Association of Blood Banks (AABB) will regulate all activities surrounding storage, handling, and administration of blood and blood products. You would be wise to review the orientation expectations of these organizations as well; however, you will likely note significant overlap between their orientation-specific guidelines and those of CMS and TJC. Ancillary regulatory bodies to consider may include:

- American Association of Blood Banks (AABB)
- College of American Pathologists (CAP)
- Commission on the Accreditation of Rehabilitation Facilities (CARF)
- American College of Surgeons, Commission on Cancer (CoC)

The only difference may be excellence awards (like the ANCC Magnet designation) that designate organizations as achieving more than the minimum standards. Requirements for these external agencies will be much higher than other regulatory bodies.

Government (Legal) Issues

Once again, working with accrediting bodies is a voluntary process to receive a designation associated with privileges. In contrast, government (legal) issues are mandatory. We want to share some legal concerns with you that relate to the orientation and onboarding process of new employees. These include:

- Licensure and certification
- Employment laws
- Occupational safety standards
- Working with your Human Resources department

Licensure and Certification

Many people get the terms *license* and *certificate* confused.

- A *license* is a government-issued document that allows you to perform certain tasks once you meet certain qualifications. Take a driver's license for example. A driver's license is issued from the state government where you are a resident once you have passed a written and driving exam. Once you have the license, you are permitted to operate certain vehicles. Similarly, a nursing license is issued by the state's board of nursing to individuals who have received an academic nursing degree and passed a national exam.

- A *certificate* is offered by governmental *or* non-governmental entities and recognizes additional accomplishment or an expanded scope of practice beyond licensure. For example, additional accomplishment is demonstrated when a public health nurse has worked in a public health setting for a certain number of hours and passes a national exam. The nurse still maintains his/her same licensure but is now also certified.

Regarding scope of practice expansion, many states do not provide a nurse practitioner *license* but rather a *certificate*. In those states, nurse practitioners still practice under their RN licenses.

Licensure is required to independently care for patients as an RN (and in many situations, even before starting orientation); certification is not. Someone in the organization should be verifying licensure through methods appropriate for that state. This is known as primary source verification and is more commonly being performed online.

During a new hire's orientation and onboarding process, the new employee should be exposed to the appropriate scope of practice for that state. You should be able to easily access the nurse practice act for your state to assist the new employee with this. You may also want to be aware of some components of the practice acts from the Board of Medicine and Board of Pharmacy to help illustrate what is *outside* the scope of practice for a nurse.

Key Employment Laws That Impact Onboarding

Several key employment laws could impact your new nurse's onboarding process. They include:

- Americans with Disabilities Act (ADA)

- Family and Medical Leave Act (FMLA)

- Pregnancy Discrimination Act (PDA)

- Title VII of the Civil Rights Act (Title VII)

- Fair Labor Standards Act (FLSA)

Let's look at these one at a time.

Americans with Disabilities Act (ADA)

The Americans with Disabilities Act (ADA) protects people with disabilities, those perceived to have disabilities, as well as employees who are associated with someone with disabilities (U.S. Equal Employment Opportunity Commission, 2013b). The U.S. Equal Employment Opportunity Commission (EEOC) oversees violations of the ADA. The EEOC has a special page designated for the ADA and healthcare workers. We suggest that you look at http://www.eeoc.gov/facts/health_care_workers.html for more information.

So, how does ADA impact you with your new employees? Well, there could be several ways. Consider these potential scenarios.

REAL-WORLD EXAMPLE: ADA SCENARIO #1

Jolene has been hired and tells you right away that she has vision issues and requires reasonable accommodation. What do you do?

1. *First, ensure that the hiring manager and Human Resources were aware of the issue before Jolene was hired.*

2. *Second, have Human Resources determine what Jolene needs in terms of reasonable accommodation.*

3. *Third, evaluate Jolene working with her reasonable accommodation as you would any other new nurse.*

Jolene is working the night shift on a unit where the modus operandi is to leave the overhead lights off when checking on patients. Jolene is accommodated with a flashlight that allows her to check vitals, etc., without disturbing the patient with overhead lights.

REAL-WORLD EXAMPLE: ADA SCENARIO #2

Fred starts onboarding and you notice that he seems to have difficulty hearing patients, their families, and you. This concerns you because you also notice that he is challenged when listening for respiration and heart sounds. What do you do?

1. *First, talk with Fred and see if he mentions any hearing issues.*

2. *Regardless of his answer, talk with his hiring manager and Human Resources next. Explain your concerns to them and tell them about the conversation with Fred.*

3. *Third, Human Resources and the hiring manager should meet with Fred to discuss the issue.*

It appears that Fred does have some hearing difficulties, but not to the level of being considered hearing disabled. That said, because it is perceived that his hearing challenge impacts his ability to do his work, a reasonable accommodation should be made, as the ADA requires accommodations for people who are perceived to be disabled. A special stethoscope is provided for Fred, and you notice that his ability to hear respiration and heart sounds improves. Things seem to be improving, until several members from different patients' families complain that they have to repeat everything three or four times with Fred. One time, he brought the wrong pain medicine to a patient because he didn't hear clearly.

At this point, you work to determine whether Fred (a) understands what medicines can be used for pain or (b) did not hear the patient. You may administer a pain medication test. He passes the test, so you document that he has the cognitive knowledge. Take the situation and results to the hiring manager and Human Resources. They will determine Fred's employment status.

What are the key takeaways from these examples? First, the ADA requires that reasonable accommodations be made so that differently-abled people can do their jobs. Second, once the reasonable accommodation is provided, the person must still be able to do all the activities of the job in a safe manner. Finally, when in doubt, bring issues to the attention of the hiring manager and your Human Resources specialist.

Family and Medical Leave Act (FMLA)

The Family and Medical Leave Act (FMLA) "entitles eligible employees of covered employers to take unpaid, job-protected leave for specified family and medical reasons with continuation of group health insurance coverage under the same terms and conditions as if the employee had not taken leave. Eligible employees are entitled to:

"Twelve workweeks of leave in a 12-month period for:

- The birth of a child and to care for the newborn child within one year of birth;

- The placement with the employee of a child for adoption or foster care and to care for the newly placed child within one year of placement;

- To care for the employee's spouse, child, or parent who has a serious health condition;

- A serious health condition that makes the employee unable to perform the essential functions of his or her job;

- Any qualifying exigency arising out of the fact that the employee's spouse, son, daughter, or parent is a covered military member on 'covered active duty;' **or**

"Twenty-six workweeks of leave during a single 12-month period to care for a covered service member with a serious injury or illness if the eligible employee is the service member's spouse, son, daughter, parent, or next of kin (military caregiver leave)" (U.S. Department of Labor, 2013c).

What's the potential impact of FMLA and your new nurses? Let's take a look at a couple scenarios.

REAL-WORLD EXAMPLE: FMLA SCENARIO #1

Jeremy's partner has been diagnosed with metastatic breast cancer. She will require surgery, chemo, and reconstruction. Jeremy talks with his hiring manager and Human Resources and applies for intermittent FMLA. Unfortunately, Jeremy misses an important class on new regulations because of his partner's illness. What do you do?

Before Jeremy leaves the day before his partner's surgery, tell him, "Jeremy, I wish you and your partner the best tomorrow. Please keep us posted on her progress. You probably saw that tomorrow, we are holding a class on new regulations. Don't worry about it. As soon as you get back to the unit, I'll review the new regs with you and make sure you understand how they impact our work."

Some organizations will record these sessions so that employees who are unable to attend can still get the information. If that is not possible, work with Jeremy the next time he is present to ensure that he understands the new regulations and how they affect work on the unit.

REAL-WORLD EXAMPLE: FMLA SCENARIO #2

Reva has been missing work, and you notice that it seems to be mostly Mondays and Fridays. You hear from her friend that Reva's dad is quite ill, and she's been going to her hometown on weekends to relieve her mom. Obviously, you are concerned about Reva and her family—and her ability to complete the onboarding. What do you do?

Talk with Reva. Say, "Reva, I've noticed that you've been missing work, mostly on Mondays and Fridays. Is there something going on that I should know about?" Reva tells you and seems relieved to have told someone else at work.

You say, "Let's go talk with your manager. You and she should talk with HR about the Family and Medical Leave Act and how you can best support your family during this difficult time, as well as protect your employment."

FMLA can be challenging to manage, especially when you are trying to get an orientee ready to go solo in your unit; however, remember that it is important for the orientee to know that his or her loved one is getting the medical treatment and support he or she needs. Communication during this time is critical so that you know when the orientee is available for additional training. The orientee will work with his or her manager regarding scheduled days away, reporting that time, etc. Your focus should be making good use of the time when the orientee is available.

Pregnancy Discrimination Act (PDA)

According to the U.S. Equal Employment Opportunity Commission, "The Pregnancy Discrimination Act (PDA) forbids discrimination based on pregnancy when it comes to any aspect of employment, including hiring, firing, pay, job assignments, promotions, layoff, training, fringe benefits, such as leave and health insurance, and any other term or condition of employment" (EEOC, 2013a, para. 2).

A pregnant employee's situation may warrant coverage under ADA as well as FMLA. If you have a pregnant employee in onboarding, work closely with the hiring manager and Human Resources to ensure that you are compliant with the relevant laws. For new employees (and especially those who are new graduate nurses) who must stop their orientation and onboarding process for a period of time, it may be difficult to pick up right where they left off. Therefore, to provide these employees with an effective learning experience while also staying in compliance with federal mandates, you may want to extend their total time spent in orientation to account for this abrupt pause in the learning experience.

REAL-WORLD EXAMPLE: PDA SCENARIO #1

Chelsea is 6 months into her pregnancy when she develops preeclampsia. She tells you that her doctor has provided written documentation requesting light duty for her. What do you do?

You should talk with the hiring manager and Human Resources to ensure that Chelsea has provided the proper documentation. Her hiring manager then meets with her and explains that due to her medical situation, her onboarding will be suspended so that she can be on "light" duty and her onboarding will continue when she returns from her maternity leave. "Light" duty for someone in the onboarding phase could involve finishing any additional classes or modules necessary for completing orientation, or even performing audits or other administrative work on the unit, which could even be beneficial from a socialization perspective with her peers.

REAL-WORLD EXAMPLE: PDA SCENARIO #2

Rachel is 8 months pregnant, and her water breaks on shift. You get her over to labor and delivery and call her partner. Rachel is 4 weeks into her onboarding process. What do you do?

You buy flowers and a teddy bear and deliver them to her room! Actually, you notify her hiring manager and Human Resources. Hopefully, Rachel has filed all the necessary paperwork for her maternity leave.

Again, communication is critical. As long as the orientee is able, work the program as you would normally. When the orientee is not able, work with the hiring manager and Human Resources specialist to make the appropriate changes in duty or schedule. Finally, when the orientee returns from maternity leave, provide some time for review before getting the orientee back into full orientation mode.

Title VII of the Civil Rights Act (Title VII)

The Civil Rights Act of 1964 is a seminal piece of legislation. Title VII of that act provided for protection against discrimination due to race, color, religion, sex, or national origin. Based on additional legislation, discrimination based on age, pregnancy status, and disabilities are also prohibited (EEOC, 2013b). Check http://www.eeoc.gov/laws/statutes/titlevii.cfm for more information. In general, Title VII should not be a factor, because the law and your organization prohibit discrimination based on the categories listed and your organization may include other categories such as sexual orientation and/or gender identity. Let's look at a quick scenario under which Title VII would be applicable.

REAL-WORLD EXAMPLE: TITLE VII SCENARIO

Abdullah is a new nurse. On your first day together, he mentions that he is Muslim and needs to pray several times during his shift. What do you do?

You check with Human Resources and find a private room where Abdullah can bring his prayer mat and pray. You ask him to find you when he has finished with his prayers and then continue the onboarding process. If the timing of the prayers may have a negative impact on patient care, discussions with the employee, hiring manager, and Human Resources should be held promptly.

Fair Labor Standards Act (FLSA)

The Fair Labor Standards Act (FLSA) "establishes minimum wage, overtime pay, recordkeeping, and youth employment standards affecting employees in the private sector and in Federal, State, and local governments. Covered nonexempt workers are entitled to a minimum wage of not less than $7.25 per hour effective July 24, 2009. Overtime pay at a rate not less than one and one-half times the regular rate of pay is required after 40 hours of work in a workweek" (U.S. Department of Labor, 2013b).

So, how does this affect you when onboarding new nurses? The main concern regarding FLSA is ensuring that an hourly employee is paid for any and all time worked and his/her time must be reported in accordance with your organization's policies.

REAL-WORLD EXAMPLE: FLSA SCENARIO

Shelby is a new nurse. You have kept her busy during the shift, and it's time for her to go home. She tells you that she's going to log into the hospital's intranet and complete some regulations training tonight. What do you do?

You say, "Shelby, it's OK to look on the intranet for your schedule, but it is against hospital policy for you to complete training at home."

Shelby responds, "Why? That seems silly."

You say, "Well, because the training is mandatory, we are required by law to pay you for your time. Our policy states that you cannot work from home."

Occupational Safety and Health Administration

The Occupational Safety and Health Administration (OSHA) is a government entity that is responsible for ensuring employees are able to work in safe and healthy environments. For healthcare workers, this will include items such as blood-borne pathogen exposure, respiratory illness protection, and hazardous waste management (U.S. Department of Labor, 2013a). All new employees (not just nurses) will need safety/health training upon hire, and we recommend contacting your Human Resources department to explore what is already being covered in general orientation. If you are part of a smaller organization, you can refer directly to OSHA's website (http://www.osha.gov), as it contains many training resources for you.

Working With Human Resources

You may have noticed that Human Resources comes up a lot in this chapter. How can you best work with your Human Resources person? As a 20-year veteran of HR, Robin has a few tips. Before we start the list, the main thing to remember is that your Human Resources professional's goal is to help you, the orientee, the hiring manager, and the organization be successful. Your HR person can partner with you on hiring, orienting, retaining, disciplining, and many other situations that arise with employees. We recommend that you:

- Develop a good relationship with your Human Resources person.

- When in doubt, contact the hiring manager and Human Resources.

- Stay current on your organization's HR policies and procedures.

- Become briefly familiar with the laws and regulations laid out in this chapter. (Who knows, you might even be able to impress your friends in HR if you throw around some of their abbreviations?)

Documentation

We couldn't consider this text complete without a proper discussion of every healthcare provider's favorite part of his/her job—documentation (can you hear the sarcasm there?). Documentation of the orientation experience is important from both a regulatory perspective (to prove that all employees have had appropriate training) as well as an organizational quality perspective (to evaluate what works and doesn't work within the organization).

To illustrate its importance, consider the following two scenarios:

REAL-WORLD EXAMPLE: THE IMPORTANCE OF DOCUMENTATION #1

A major error has occurred in which a surgical patient received the procedure on the incorrect limb. The state's health department has been contacted to investigate the situation, and they want to review whether or not all employees in the operating room have been properly trained on ensuring the correct surgical site is marked.

The unit-based educators bring spreadsheets with completion dates of all regulatory and accrediting body mandatory education requirements. The auditors can verify that staff members have received the appropriate training, and further exploration of the error can continue.

REAL-WORLD EXAMPLE: THE IMPORTANCE OF DOCUMENTATION #2

Senior-level management is looking to reduce orientation length as a means for alleviating financial challenges. They have requested information regarding the average length of the current competency-based orientation. After unit-based educators retrieved orientation documentation over the last 2 years, the educators were able to provide data to management that indicated the current length is well below that of surrounding organizations and requested that orientation length not be cut. Management moved their attention to other areas to enact budget cuts.

In both scenarios, having documentation available provided evidence that the standard was being met. Without this documented data, it can be difficult (or even impossible) to demonstrate compliance and/or performance.

ESSENTIAL DOCUMENTATION

It can be difficult to determine which documents to keep and which ones to trash if you're new to the realm of orientation. To be safe, it is wise to keep more than you trash in the beginning. You can always do some "spring cleaning" once you have a better grasp on what documents are important. To help you get started, though, here are some essential documents we recommend you keep:

- *Offer letter*
- *A copy of licenses and certifications (if these cannot be immediately accessible online)*
- *Proof of orientation completion with signatures of key personnel*
- *Proof of regulatory/mandatory module and class completions*
- *Orientation schedule (along with assigned preceptor)*
- *Rental equipment/supply agreement forms (e.g., pagers, keys)*

Dos and Don'ts

To provide you with some quick action items on how to handle documentation issues, check out Table 8.2. Rationale for many of these items may be found throughout the chapter.

TABLE 8.2 Dos and Don'ts of Orientation Documentation

DO	DON'T
Have all key principals (manager, educator, preceptor, and orientee) sign competency documents.	Forget the orientees (they must verify that they have ownership of the learning process, too, and that they acknowledge receipt of all necessary learning opportunities).
Ensure the documents are easily retrievable by the appropriate personnel (managers, auditors, etc.).	Neglect security & confidentiality of documents to the degree that anybody could access the records.
Keep proof of initial competency assessment.	Keep *everything* unless it can be easily stored electronically.
Maintain organized records by either alphabetical order or date of hire.	Simply throw everything in a pile or closet (if you do, being audited will be a nightmare).
Include proof of all regulatory training requirements, especially those mandates ending with the statement "upon hire" (or the like).	Depend on the orientee nor one single person or department to keep this record (tracking at both the organizational level and the departmental level may prove beneficial).

Formatting and Medium

To our knowledge, there is no external agency that regulates what the training documents should look like. The formatting of the document and whether it is electronic or on paper is left to the discretion of each organization. As long as the documentation is easily retrievable during an audit and the manager (or his/her designee) can walk an auditor through the document, you are in good shape.

Paper documents are easier to develop and share among preceptors; however, retrieval of data can become more cumbersome (either during an audit or if the nurse transfers to a different unit in the organization where the paperwork looks different). Ornate electronic forms of documentation may not be possible in organizations with limited resources, but even relatively simple documents can be prepared with either Microsoft Word or Microsoft Excel. The benefits of these electronic forms of documentation are that they are easily searchable, and they can be shared and stored with multiple persons. If you work in a very large organization, check with the central Learning and Development (Education) department. They may have a Learning Management System (LMS) that will make it easier to track your orientees' information as well as provide necessary reports for governing and accrediting bodies.

In regard to format of the document, we want to share one example Alvin helped develop at Cincinnati Children's Hospital Medical Center. This form (Figure 8.2) is a document used throughout the organization that can be modified by each individual unit/department. The template was developed by the hospital and based on Patricia Benner's Novice to Expert continuum, the AACN Synergy Model, and the organization's job standards and clinical ladder.

Cincinnati Children's Hospital Medical Center   Name:
Department of Patient Services Nursing Services Orientation   Unit:
Core Competency Assessment Tool for Newly Hired RN's 2013   Educator:
                                                                 Preceptor:

Phases of Orientation

The 4 phases of orientation, based on Patricia's Benner's novice to expert model, defines increasing complexity of learning, and incorporates the three domains of learning and skill acquisition (cognitive learning, psychomotor skill demonstration, and affective reasoning). The increasing complexity is noted in the expected behaviors supporting each competency statement and phase.

The phases of orientation Is a behavior based approach. It provides that the nurse may progress through orientation based on assessment of demonstrated expected behaviors ensuring competent practice rather than solely on time.

The newly hired RN progresses through orientation with Preceptor Assistance, Preceptor Guidance and then to independent practice with Preceptor as Resource.

Requires manager, educator, preceptor and orientee to meet and sign off as each phase is completed.

Phase I: Weeks 1 and 2 of Orientation   (Education Consultant/Orientation Facilitator Guided)

Phase II: Assimilation   (Preceptor Assistance)
> *Preceptor is present and actively supports orientee with learning opportunities.*
> *Preceptor teaches and assesses practice of new orientee.*

Phase III: Adaptation   (Preceptor Guidance)
> *Preceptor facilitates learning; maximizes learning opportunities.*
> *Preceptor encourages orientee to identify learning needs.*

Phase IV: Synthesis   (Preceptor as a Resource)
> *Preceptor familiar with orientee's experiences and is available as a resource when needed.*

Continues

Cincinnati Children's Hospital Medical Center
Department of Patient Services Nursing Services Orientation
Core Competency Assessment Tool for Newly Hired RN's 2013

Name:
Unit:
Educator:
Preceptor:

Environment of Care: Socialization to Unit Environment

Introduce the orientee to the team and key resource people on the unit. Use huddle and rounds as opportunities for the orientee to understand how the team works together on your unit. Make sure that the new staff member learns not only about the layout of the unit but also the unit culture. Set up times to meet on a regular basis. Include the educator and manager at least every 2 weeks. Create an environment where the orientee feels safe to ask questions or express concerns.

Validation Statement	Verification/Source of Evaluation
☐ Demonstrates familiarity with unit resources.	Supported by:
☐ Demonstrates awareness of emergency preparedness resources.	☐ Completion of Learning Opportunities
☐ Demonstrates awareness of parent and guest support services.	

Opportunities		
Introduction to Roles and Responsibilities **HealthCare Team Members**	**Finding your way** ☐ Breakroom, restrooms, lockers	**Parent/Guest Support Services**
☐ Director/Managers	☐ Medication room/medication refrigerator	☐ Laundry Facilities
☐ Charge RN	☐ Huddle Room	☐ Parent Meals
☐ RNs	☐ Child life	☐ Family /Visitor Guidelines
☐ PCA	☐ Tub/shower room	☐ Family Relations
☐ HUC	☐ Kitchen	**Introduction to unit specific Guidelines/Resources**
☐ Care Coordinator	☐ Dirty utility room	☐ Staffing guidelines
☐ Educator	☐ Dirty tube system	☐ Scheduling process
☐ Environmental Care		☐ Holiday requirements/rotation

Cincinnati Children's Hospital Medical Center
Department of Patient Services Nursing Services Orientation
Core Competency Assessment Tool for Newly Hired RN's 2013

Name:
Unit:
Educator:
Preceptor:

NURSING PROCESS   **Validation Statements**

Phase II Assimilation Demonstrates initial competence in development and use of the *NURSING PROCESS*	**Phase III Adaptation** Demonstrates development and use of the *NURSING PROCESS*	**Phase IV Synthesis** Demonstrates independent development and use of the *NURSING PROCESS*
Completes appropriate assessment for each Body System. ☐ Respiratory; Cardiovascular; Endocrine; Genitourinary; Gastrointestinal/Nutritional Status; Head, Ear, Eye, Nose and Throat (HEENT); Integumentary; Musculoskeletal; Neuro/Psychiatric; Reproductive ☐ Correlates assessment findings from patient care equipment with the physical assessment findings/clinical picture. Treats the patient, not the machine. ☐ Identifies normal/abnormal findings (Physical, diagnostic testing, vital signs, I&O's, psychosocial and discusses that information with the preceptor.	☐ Incorporate the nursing process; prioritize care based upon an assessment continuum. ☐ Create a plan of care integrating all aspects of clinical findings and assessments. ☐ Perform admissions, transfers, and/or discharges with preceptor guidance. ☐ Apply growth and development concepts, cultural considerations and psychosocial needs for patients and families throughout the nursing process. ☐ Demonstrate ability to locate CCHMC/department resources related to nursing interventions.	☐ Consistent use of the nursing process; prioritizes care based upon an assessment continuum. ☐ Anticipate potential problems and identify potential solutions. ☐ Independently perform admissions, transfers, and/or discharges. ☐ Consistently apply growth and development concepts, cultural considerations and psychosocial needs for patients and families. ☐ Utilize appropriate resources related to nursing interventions. ☐ Evaluate performance management RN job responsibilities.

Continues

Cincinnati Children's Hospital Medical Center
Department of Patient Services Nursing Services Orientation
Core Competency Assessment Tool for Newly Hired RN's 2013

Name:
Unit:
Educator:
Preceptor:

Learning Opportunities for *NURSING PROCESS*

Assessment/Evaluation
- ☐ Care for __ number of types of patients specific to unit/clinic subspecialty population.
- ☐ Participates in admission/discharge transfer process
- ☐ Standard Precautions / Isolation Precautions/PPE
- ☐ Rounds /huddles
- ☐ Fall Risk Assessment
- ☐ Pain Assessment
- ☐ Catheter Associated Urinary Tract Infection Prevention Bundle CA-UTI
- ☐ PIV Catheter Care and IV Assessment
- ☐ CVC and PIV Extravasation and Grading
- ☐ Situational Awareness (e.g. watcher, family concern, PEWS)
- ☐ Vital signs
- ☐ Adult Patient Care

Emergency Care
- ☐ Change of Shift Bedside Safety Check
- ☐ Suction Equipment (presence & set up)
- ☐ Portable Suction
- ☐ Oxygen Set Up
- ☐ Portable Oxygen Cylinders
- ☐ Code Button / Panic Button / Staff Assist
- ☐ Code Sheets
- ☐ Call light functions
- ☐ Crash Cart/Defibrillator
- ☐ Safe environment (e.g. bed placement, side rails up, nurse server locked)

Equipment/Devices
Patient Monitor
- ☐ Dash®
- ☐ Solar®

CCHMC Resource: Equipment How-To & JIT aids (Mosby)
Oxygen Delivery Methods
- ☐ Nasal Cannula
- ☐ Simple Mask

Anthropometrics
- ☐ Standing Scale
- ☐ Infant Scale

Cincinnati Children's Hospital Medical Center
Department of Patient Services Nursing Services Orientation
Core Competency Assessment Tool for Newly Hired RN's 2013

Name:
Unit:
Educator:
Preceptor:

Notes on Progress Page: This page can be used for documentation by preceptor, educator, and a peer for "just in time" Learning opportunities that the newly hired RN experiences day to day. Notes can include Number of patients assigned /ages of patient / diagnosis / skills and procedures / equipment and devices etc.
In addition, the newly hired RN must be aware of resources and demonstrate ability to access resources in the face of uncertainty. Documentation of examples of how the newly hired RN demonstrates expected Safety behaviors and supporting techniques can be captured on the Notes Progress page.

Preceptor Initials / Date:	Age of Pt:	Type of Pt / Diagnosis:
Notes on Demonstrated Safety Behaviors/ Skills Performed / Equipment Training:		

Preceptor Initials / Date:	Age of Pt:	Type of Pt / Diagnosis:
Notes on Demonstrated Safety Behaviors/ Skills Performed / Equipment Training:		

Cincinnati Children's Hospital Medical Center
Department of Patient Services Nursing Services Orientation
Core Competency Assessment Tool for Newly Hired RN's 2013

Name:
Unit:
Educator:
Preceptor:

Orientation Guideline Phases Completion

Phase II
☐ The components of Phase II are either complete or have been addressed by the preceptor and orientee.
Preceptor Signature: _____   Date: _____
Educator signature: _____   Date: _____
Manager/Director signature: _____   Date: _____

Phase III
☐ The components of Phase III are either complete or have been addressed by the preceptor and orientee.
Preceptor Signature: _____   Date: _____
Educator signature: _____   Date: _____
Manager/Director signature: _____   Date: _____

Phase IV
☐ The components of Phase IV are either complete or have been addressed by the preceptor and orientee.
Preceptor Signature: _____   Date: _____
Educator signature: _____   Date: _____
Manager/Director signature: _____   Date: _____
Orientee signature: _____   Date: _____

Verification/Source of Evaluation
Supported by:
☐ *Completion of Learning Opportunities*

☐ *Skills Checklist*

☐ *Module with Post Test*

Verified by:
☐ *Evidence of Daily Practice*

☐ *Peer/preceptor Assessment*

☐ *Educator Assessment*

☐ *Documentation Review*

Comments:

FIGURE 8.2
Example of a competency document.

What to Keep, Where to Keep It, and How Long to Keep It

Determining what documents to keep can be very overwhelming, especially for new educators and managers. There is a tendency to keep too many things when first starting in the new position to make sure you have all your bases covered. If you start your process by looking up all the appropriate regulatory guidelines and keep track of what they request be documented, you'll be in good shape. Try to place yourself in their shoes and ask yourself, "If I were the auditor, what would I need to see to ensure the organization has provided appropriate training of all new employees in [insert topic: e.g., restraints]?"

To help with this, consider attaching the source statement of a regulatory requirement to your competency assessment spreadsheet so that others will know *why* you are tracking certain items. In organizations where nurse leaders frequently change positions, it can be helpful for incoming leaders to see the source statement of a requirement rather than depending on anecdotal stories.

Regarding location of orientation competency documentation, the unit educator may be able to keep documents in his/her office throughout the orientation and onboarding period. Once the new employee has completed the onboarding process (or if a regulatory body performs an audit), all documents should be sent to the manager, who can then forward necessary documents to Human Resources. The reason the manager should have the easiest access to the documents is because the manager (or his/her designee) is the one ultimately responsible for competency assessment according to most regulatory bodies.

Evidence of initial competency assessment should probably be retained for the duration of an individual's employment in that unit or department. For more general topics (such as patient rights, cultural diversity, etc.), completion documentation should be retained throughout the individual's employment with the organization. Ongoing competency assessment can be destroyed after 3 to 6 years (depending on the particular regulatory body's requirements); however, initial competency records should be retained. This does not necessarily mean that, for example, a 10-page medication quiz must be retained in the employee's record; however, evidence of taking the quiz and passing it (perhaps along with the score) should be placed in writing in the orientation record. Compiling all orientation-related documentation into one folder to place into the employee's personnel file will help keep that record organized and easily retrievable.

Confidentiality

Orientation records, like other personnel records, should remain as confidential as possible. Especially if there were issues during an employee's orientation period that could result in embarrassment for the individual, confidentiality of information should be protected. The manager, orientee, and Human Resources personnel should be the only employees with unlimited access to the personnel record.

Educators likely will have access to most of the orientation record. An exception would be the example of an orientee who must take a medical leave during the orientation period. The manager and Human Resources can work with the orientee on the reason for the leave, but the educator only needs to know when the leave will occur so that scheduling of appropriate learning activities can occur. The orientee can share this information with the educator, if desired, but the educator does not need access to this information to carry out his/her duties.

Preceptors will need access to a significant portion of the orientation records to carry out their teaching duties. For example, they may need to see preferred learning styles, learning activities already completed, and areas for improvement. They will not need as much access as the educator and manager, but it will be important to keep them in the loop if they are to create a highly effective learning atmosphere.

Other than the orientee, manager, Human Resources, educator, and preceptors, no other employees should need access to information found in the new employee's orientation record. Protecting this information through the use of physical locks or password-protected files will help to guarantee employee privacy and offset organizational liability.

NOTE

Regarding documentation, confidentiality, etc.—when in doubt, check with the hiring manager and your Human Resources professional.

Conclusion

The abundance of accrediting and legal guidelines can be overwhelming, especially if you don't have much time to explore them on your own. However, the time spent retrieving source statements and becoming familiar with what's actually required will yield a significant return on your investment. We highly recommend taking a day or two to become familiar with all the various requirements and organize them for yourself. If you can organize the orientation-related requirements and then document compliance with all of them, when the auditors come around, you'll have no reason for anxiety.

Questions for Reflection/Discussion

1. What are your greatest fears or challenges regarding regulatory or accrediting bodies?

2. What are possible action steps you could take to become more prepared for a regulatory body or accrediting body audit?

3. What are the strengths and weaknesses of your current approach to documentation of orientation competency assessment?

KEY TAKEAWAYS

- *As healthcare workers, it is critical to stay current on relevant regulatory changes.*

- *Since you are working with orientees, you must stay current on relevant labor laws as well.*

- *Recordkeeping is important to your success and the continued compliance of your organization.*

- *When in doubt, contact your Human Resources liaison.*

References

Centers for Medicare and Medicaid Services (CMS). (2015). *State operations manual*. Retrieved from http://www.cms.gov/ Regulations-and-Guidance/Guidance/Manuals/downloads/ som107ap_a_hospitals.pdf

The Joint Commission. (2017). *The Joint Commission manual*. Released July 1, 2017. Retrieved from http://www.jointcommission.org/

U.S. Department of Labor. (2013a). Occupational Safety and Health Administration, Clinicians. Retrieved from https://www.osha.gov/ dts/oom/clinicians/index.html

U.S. Department of Labor. (2013b). Wage and Hour Division (WHD), Compliance assistance—Wages and the Fair Labor Standards Act (FLSA). Retrieved from http://www.dol.gov/whd/flsa/

U.S. Department of Labor. (2013c). Wage and Hour Division (WHD), Family and Medical Leave Act. Retrieved from http://www.dol.gov/ whd/fmla/

U.S. Equal Employment Opportunity Commission (EEOC). (2013a). Pregnancy discrimination. Retrieved from http://www.eeoc.gov/ laws/types/pregnancy.cfm

U.S. Equal Employment Opportunity Commission (EEOC). (2013b). Title VII of the Civil Rights Act of 1964. Retrieved from http:// www.eeoc.gov/laws/statutes/titlevii.cfm

CHAPTER 9

Practical Tips for Staying Organized

Introduction

We hope you've found all the previous content helpful and insightful, but if you're new to managing orientation and onboarding programs, we expect you might be feeling a little overwhelmed at this point. You might even be thinking, "I don't care about improving the system. I just need to be able to keep my head above water!" This chapter is devoted to offering practical tips and examples of how to stay organized.

Why are we devoting a whole chapter to such a basic concept? Well, there are several reasons. Alvin's experience in training new educators has been that even though they have lots of great ideas and enthusiasm, those can quickly be stifled once the number of responsibilities and tasks pile up into a seemingly insurmountable challenge. Additionally, nursing school taught you how to organize patient care, but there was probably no mention of how to organize your office schedule or your email inbox. And, if you are the first professional development specialist your unit has had, there is likely no one to tell you how to organize your orientees' information.

Communication Strategies

Although interoffice and postal mail are still options for communicating with others, email and phone calls are probably your most utilized communication strategies. Their ease of use, though, has contributed to a significant increase in the number of messages sent and received on a daily basis, and organizing all of these messages can be quite overwhelming. We want to offer you a few strategies to help you keep these messages organized.

Email

In today's healthcare world, email will most likely be the primary way you communicate with others. Because of this, you really want to keep your email messages organized. Having thousands of messages in your inbox will make it difficult to find emails easily and to stay organized. Additionally, most Information Technology (IT) departments have set a limit to the size your inbox can be—you will have to file those emails eventually! If you do it as messages come in, your life will be much easier.

Some email programs allow you to "flag" or "mark" the message as being high-priority or even automatically add it to a to-do list. This is a great way to get started. Some people will keep the message marked as "unread" if it's a high-priority email. Regardless of how you mark the important messages, once you have responded to or taken care of the request, you should move the message out of your inbox. You can move it to another folder if you want to keep it for later, but at least move it out of your inbox. You will be surprised at how much of a relief it can be to have an email inbox that can display all messages on one page, rather than having to scroll to find a message.

Probably the best advice for keeping your email messages organized is to create folders and subfolders for storing messages. Every person prefers a slightly different system, but Figure 9.1 demonstrates one option to consider. You could have a folder for every orientee or a folder for every cohort, or both. Additionally, in managing orientation activities, you probably want a folder for each class, activity, or committee in which you participate (see Figure 9.2). If you think a message fits into two categories, you could consider forwarding it to yourself (so that you have a total of two copies) and place one in each desired folder. Some email programs, such as Microsoft Outlook, will allow you to copy a message and place it in the additional folder.

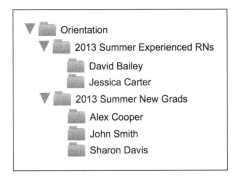

FIGURE 9.1

Methods for organizing orientees into folders and subfolders.

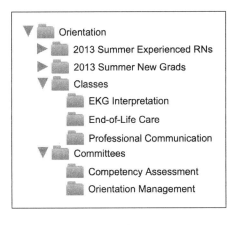

FIGURE 9.2

Methods for organizing orientation activities into folders and subfolders.

Some people prefer to skip meticulous folder management in favor of searching for messages based on a keyword. This can work too, unless the message happens not to contain the keyword you search. For example, if you were looking for all the confidentiality agreements from new hires during the past year, and you search for "confidentiality," you would not retrieve messages in which the new hire simply said, "Here's my agreement." By having a folder devoted to confidentiality agreements, you would know where all of them were located. Given the amount of information most of us receive on a daily basis, we would not recommend the keyword approach. You will save yourself a lot of time and pain by using a folder system.

If you will not have access to email for several days (yes, you should still take vacations even if you are in charge of orientation), you would be wise to set up an automatic reply message that will inform the sender of when you expect to have access to email again and whom he/she could contact if there is an immediate need. Also, before going on vacation, your email program may allow you to set up "Rules" that would forward certain emails to a special folder, so that your inbox does not become too unwieldy while you're gone. Rules in the email program can be useful any time, but particularly when you're away from the office.

Phone

Whether you have an office phone, a mobile phone, a pager, or even all three, this will be an important method for staying organized. Especially if you have a smartphone as your mobile phone, you can get additional information like emails, calendar appointments, and even to-do lists. Contact your IT department for assistance in setting this up.

Even if you don't have a smartphone, make sure your phone has a professional voicemail message for when you are unavailable to answer your phone. Additionally, if you go on an extended leave, set an out-of-office message with details of when you'll return to the office and whom the caller can contact if he/she has an urgent need.

TIP

If you'd like to take advantage of smartphone applications for staying organized and communicating with orientees (or anyone involved in structured orientation activities), you might consider app-based, formal messaging systems (e.g., Remind [available at https://www.remind.com]). These messaging systems allow you to send out reminders to mobile phones or communicate last-minute changes (e.g., a room change for a class beginning in the next hour). Using a service like this also prevents you from giving out your mobile phone number (which is frequently a personal phone number) to your learners.

Managing a Calendar

Maintaining an accurate calendar is essential to staying organized. Whether it's meetings with administrators and new hires, teaching a class, or simply making time for lunch on a busy day, knowing where to be and when is key to meeting all your responsibilities. The simple part of maintaining a calendar is writing things down when you get invited to a meeting (or if details get changed). The more complex part starts when you begin scheduling the details of a major task.

Plan Ahead!

Although calendars can be useful to help you organize your day as soon as you get into the office, the real time-management benefit will be seen in planning ahead...days, weeks, and even months ahead! Let's take the practical example of sending a new hire through orientation and onboarding. When a new person starts, you want to place every possible meeting on the calendar, and then reschedule if needed. If it doesn't make it to the calendar in advance, it may never make it.

Table 9.1 has a timeline of potential activities and meetings to place in your calendar when a new employee starts. As soon as you discover a new employee is starting, we recommend placing all of these events on your calendar in one sitting to make sure you don't leave anything out. However, you may have to wait until you have more details about the orientee's unit-level schedule before planning exact times. If you don't have all the details at the beginning, you could consider placing timed reminders or to-do items at the beginning of the week to provide you with a cue to confirm an appropriate time.

Obviously, this is just a rough sketch, and you are encouraged to meet with the new employee more frequently than this table recommends. Hopefully you can see how complex a calendar might become if you have multiple new hires in orientation at the same time. By placing all significant dates on your calendar as soon as you can predict them, you are more likely to stay on track. These frequent meetings with the new employee will also demonstrate to the employee that you care about his/her performance.

TABLE 9.1 Activities to Place in Calendar When a New Employee Starts

Background: You are the unit-based educator in a medical-surgical unit where orientation typically lasts 8 weeks, and the centralized educators are responsible for scheduling general hospital and nursing orientation. Your manager has just informed you that a new nurse will be starting 4 weeks from now.

TIME	ACTIVITY
4 Weeks Pre-Hire	Place new hire's start date on your calendar.
2 Weeks Pre-Hire	Schedule phone call (~15 min.) to talk with orientee and gather more information.
Week 1	Meet face-to-face with new employee during central orientation (consider scheduling a lunch meeting that includes managers and preceptors).
	Schedule at least 1 hour to provide new employee with a tour of the unit and other activities needed before taking care of patients.
Week 2/3	Schedule at least 15 minutes to simply check on the orientee and preceptor.
Week 4	Schedule meeting with manager, preceptor, and orientee to formally evaluate mid-orientation progress.
Week 5/6	Schedule at least 15 minutes to simply check on the orientee and preceptor.
Week 7/8	Mark orientee's tentative last day.
	Schedule meeting with manager, preceptor, and orientee to formally evaluate orientation progress and determine readiness for practicing independently.
Immediately Post-Orientation	Schedule at least 15 minutes on several days to check on independent orientee.
90 Days Post-Hire	Place a "Probationary Evaluation Due" item on calendar.

TIP

As an alternative to a traditional individual-focused calendar, you might consider creating a Gantt chart for yourself so you can monitor multiple, overlapping orientees at the same time. Gantt charts visually display the start and end of large tasks and their sub-tasks. You can find templates within electronic spreadsheet software (e.g., Microsoft Excel) or on websites (e.g., dapulse [available at https://www.dapulse.com]).

Paper vs. Electronic

Some people prefer paper calendars rather than electronic versions. But in today's healthcare environment, an electronic calendar is almost a necessity. Some people like to have both available (e.g., the electronic calendar is for work and the paper calendar is for family), but be careful when adding events because you don't want to double-book yourself. In many electronic calendars, you can mark appointments as confidential or private so that others cannot see your personal appointments. You also have the ability to apply different color schemes to different types of appointments, so you can easily see what is a work-related meeting versus what is your kid's soccer game. Consider syncing your calendar with your smartphone or other portable device. Because most people always have their phones with them, a paper calendar will be one less thing to remember to have on hand.

Other benefits of having an electronic version of your calendar include:

- Accessible anywhere with a network connection

- Others can view or modify your calendar if they have permission to do so

- Invitations from others can easily be added to your calendar

- Frequent changes will not result in a "messy" look

- Easier to set up meetings with others who also have an electronic calendar

- Search function typically available

- Forward calendar events and invitations to others who need to attend

- Can add repetitive events (such as weekly or monthly meetings) quickly

Even though we recommend going paperless to stay organized, there is still benefit in having paper (or sticky notes) available. You will find something that works for you, but until then, try experimenting with different methods.

Ongoing Review of Orientation/Onboarding Program

We've mentioned the use of the ADDIE model throughout this book. Because this is a cycle intended to be repeated (and because the needs of the organization change regularly), you should set aside time for regular review of various aspects of your orientation and onboarding program. You should schedule these reviews far in advance for a couple reasons:

1. Ensuring the presence of key stakeholders for high-level program analysis and evaluation

2. Maintaining up-to-date learning activities

For the high-level program analysis and evaluation, you may want to consider scheduling a standing annual meeting with key stakeholders. By scheduling a meeting far in advance (up to a year), you can increase your chances that all the desired people will be there. From the perspective of current learning activities, you could schedule annual reviews of classes and modules by subject-matter experts. Some organizations change so frequently that learning activities (especially those without a facilitator) may quickly become outdated, and you want to be certain new employees are receiving a relevant learning experience.

You also may want to set aside an hour each quarter to check for regulatory or other changes that affect your onboarding and orientation program. In addition to the annual review with key stakeholders, this will help ensure that your program stays up-to-date—and legal!

Computer Folders

For your dedicated work computer, you may want to place shortcuts on the desktop that link to your most commonly used folders and files. Especially when accessing files that are stored in subfolders of a shared/network drive, you can waste a lot of time searching for files. So, instead of clicking through multiple folders to get to a destination, place a hyperlink or shortcut in an easily accessible location. This could be on your desktop, or you could have a spreadsheet or text document that has embedded hyperlinks to desired files.

Once you've been managing orientation and onboarding projects for a few months, you will probably have several files on your computer that you are particularly fond of and have spent a lot of time perfecting. The last thing you want is for your hard drive to go bad and lose this information. Consider the following methods for having an extra copy available for a rainy day:

- Email a copy of the file to yourself

- Store a copy on a thumb drive or external hard drive

- Create a backup folder in the "cloud" or on your organization's server

- Regularly back up your local hard drive

You might also consider moving a lot of your files to a server or cloud-based location so that documents can be accessed and shared more easily (in addition to the peace of mind that comes with knowing your files won't be lost in a hard-drive crash). Your organization's IT department might be able to set up shared folders for you, or you could consider moving data into the cloud. Products such as Dropbox, Google Drive, and Microsoft OneDrive offer the ability to access files remotely and collaborate easily with others. These functions can be helpful when you're teaching a class offsite and forget your flash drive, you want to work on a presentation with an educator in another department, or you want to share materials with learners without printing a lot of handouts.

TIP

Another tool that is helpful is Microsoft OneNote. OneNote allows you to keep all your electronic files in one overall file. Excel spreadsheets, Word documents, PowerPoint slides, notes to yourself—accessible to you, all in one convenient file! You might want to consider several OneNote files or just one really big one—it's up to you. You could organize the OneNote files by cohort group or by administration (planning, budgeting, etc.) versus cohort (orientees' information).

Spreadsheets

Whether you're responsible for 5 employees or 500, maintaining an organized, easily searchable record of all relevant dates for orientation and competencies is an essential role of the educator and/ or manager. Most people will use some sort of spreadsheet to organize this information because you can search the spreadsheet for desired information and organize the information into reports, and because data input is relatively simple. Some organizations will create databases instead of keeping all information in spreadsheets, but database creation and management is a complex project that is beyond the scope of most nursing professional development specialists.

This section is not intended to replace the "Help" function in your software but rather to point you in the direction of some features specific to the role of a professional development specialist. If you're using Microsoft Excel and want a few extra tips, Alvin recommends *101 Excel 2013 Tips, Tricks & Timesavers,* by John Walkenbach (John Wiley & Sons, 2013).

Our recommendations for designing effective spreadsheets can be found in Table 9.2. Several of these recommendations are represented in Figures 9.3, 9.4, and 9.5.

TABLE 9.2 Spreadsheet Recommendations

RECOMMENDATION	RATIONALE
Place only one word or date in each column (e.g., have a column for "First Name" and "Last Name" rather than just "Name")	This allows for filtering based on specific criteria and prevents inconsistencies in data input.
Use "Comments" for adding qualitative data	Most additional qualitative information is unique to that entry, so a separate column isn't necessary.
Consider placing a unique identifier (e.g., employee ID) in the far-left column	Facilitates integration of spreadsheet data into a database should that be necessary in the future. Also necessary for "VLOOKUP" formulas, if desired.
Add color to spreadsheet	Color makes the spreadsheet easier to read.
Create a copy of the spreadsheet every year (e.g., "Education Spreadsheet 2012")	Keeps data succinct, as more education requirements are added or changed each year. Prevents loss of all data in the event of file corruption.
Add an "AutoFilter" toward the top of the spreadsheet	Provides easy ability to sort by items such as name, date completed, or even missing data.
Divide spreadsheet or workbook into smaller worksheets that are functional (e.g., by cohort or discipline)	Having a functional organization to a spreadsheet can assist with rapid retrieval of desired information.

	B	C	D	E	F	G
1	Last Name	First Name	Hire Date	Completed Orientation	CPR Expiration	Glucose Meter
3	Brodeur	Susan	7/29/08	9/30/08	11/29/13	7/28/13
4	Clark	Dena	6/8/90	8/8/90	2/21/14	7/26/13
5	France	Debra	10/13/96	12/10/96	9/23/14	7/25/13
6	Jarvis	David	11/9/88	1/9/89	11/7/13	7/27/13
7	Jeffery	Bill	8/11/99	10/11/99	2/3/14	7/14/13
8	Mueller	Beth	1/4/08	3/1/08	8/7/13	7/23/13
9	Rutschilling	Jamey	5/13/12	7/13/12	2/25/13	7/9/13

FIGURE 9.3

Example spreadsheet.

Figure 9.3 is an example of a basic spreadsheet where we have listed all of the employees' names along with significant dates. Although we have only listed hire date, orientation completion date, and a few educational requirements, you could place any and all relevant dates into a spreadsheet. The second row (immediately under the heading row) is a blank row with a filter added. These filters (displayed by arrows) allow you to sort the data in various ways (e.g., placing the information in ascending order by hire date to determine who has the most tenure). In the example listed here, the data are filtered and sorted by last name, so that employees are easily listed in alphabetical order.

	A	B	C	D	E
1	Employee ID	Last Name	First Name	Hire Date	Completed Orient:
3	38729	Brodeur	Susan	7/29/08	
4	24372	Clark	Dena	6/8/90	Author: Did not start with the
5	65983	France	Debra	10/13/96	rest of her cohort.

FIGURE 9.4

Use of unique identifier and comments.

Figure 9.4 has the same information as Figure 9.3 but with the addition of a unique employee identifier. Placing this column on the far left is recommended if you hope to integrate the information into a database (or intend on using a VLOOKUP function). The other addition to this figure is the presence of a comment. After a comment is added to a cell, if you move your mouse over the cell, a pop-up box will appear with the contents of the comment (in this case, the comment box states "Did not start with the rest of her cohort.").

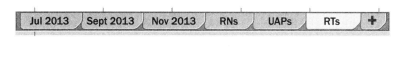

FIGURE 9.5
Use of worksheets (tabs).

Figure 9.5 illustrates the creation of several worksheets (tabs). Each of these tabs, once clicked, will display a different worksheet within the same workbook (file). The three tabs on the left of this figure demonstrate the organization of new employee cohorts based on their hire date, and the three tabs on the right are organized based on discipline/profession of the new hires.

Learning Management System (LMS)

If you work in a large organization and have a centralized Training and Development (T&D) department, this department may have purchased a learning management system (LMS). The department should be delighted if you approach them and want to track your orientees' progress on the LMS. You will want to work with the T&D folks to set up the classes and experiences in a way that makes it easy for you to track and is consistent with the structure the T&D department uses. This makes tracking and reporting a whole lot easier.

If you don't have an LMS in your organization, you may want to consider getting one. Even with an initial start-up cost, you may quickly begin saving money if your time is devoted to *teaching* as opposed to *tracking*. Many companies specialize in LMS development, and you could contact one of their representatives or search for information online if you want more information about what they are able to offer. Some questions you want to ask before purchasing a new LMS may include:

- Can we design courses to be housed in the LMS, or is it simply for tracking purposes?

- What are options for data input and data output (e.g., manual and automatic)?

- Can reports be customized?
- Is there a one-time cost or an annual fee (or both)?
- How much do updates and improvements cost?
- Does the system integrate with other systems, such as performance management?
- What kind of technical assistance and training is available?

Many learning management systems are now available in the cloud, so they don't take a lot of internal IT support. That said, you still need to work with your IT group to implement any type of LMS. You will not want an open-source system, as it may be difficult to protect the confidentiality of your participants and their results.

Here are some LMS's that might meet your needs. Please note that these are not recommendations but rather a partial list to get started in exploring LMS's!

- Saba—http://www.saba.com/us
- Success Factors—http://www.successfactors.com/
- TrainCaster—http://www.traincaster.com/index.html
- Blackboard—http://www.blackboard.com/Platforms.aspx
- HealthStream—http://www.healthstream.com
- Cornerstone On Demand—http://www.cornerstoneondemand.com

Paper Documentation

Some of you may not have all the technology available to you that we have discussed in this chapter. That's fine; we have ideas to help you, too! There are ways to organize your paper documentation as well.

- If you have orientees in a cohort, you should consider keeping all their paper documentation in a notebook marked with the start date. You should then keep their documentation by type (such as confidentiality agreements) in alphabetical order.

- If you don't have cohorts, keep paper files on each new hire, and keep those in alphabetical order. On the orientee's file folder label, you might note hire date. This can help you easily access your files when someone asks to see information on people hired on a certain date.

- You might decide to organize by type of training or documentation. If you do that, we would recommend that you use subcategories by date and then alphabetize by last name.

Records Retention

Your organization may have some policies or guidelines about records retention. Just like you should keep your tax returns for at least 7 years, there are guidelines about how long you need to keep certain types of records (paper and electronic). Please check with the records retention person to find out what you need to keep and for how long. Chapter 8 also touches on this topic.

Building and Maintaining a Budget

Building and maintaining a budget will demonstrate to management that you understand money doesn't grow on trees and that you are willing to be objective in the distribution (and potentially the evaluation) of funds. You may not get all the money that you want (few people do), but by outlining the items you deem important along with their cost, you have an objective product to help facilitate discussions. The final approval will be in the hands of the manager, but as the subject matter expert, you are the best person to know what to ask for. Consider placing the following items in your budget:

- Orientee salary (although this is typically already included in organizational budgets)

- Teaching materials (books, office supplies, patient care equipment, software)

- Laptop and projector

- Camera

- Patient simulator and/or manikin

- Professional development materials (such as buying books or attending a conference for your development)

Conclusion

We don't expect that you implement everything like we have it here, but we hope you've learned a couple tips or gained a few ideas for getting (or staying) organized. Many of these skills and techniques are not something you would learn in nursing school or even during the orientation period to a new leadership role. Unfortunately, these are also the skills that can make your role very frustrating if you don't acquire them. In addition to what we have listed here, don't be afraid to perform a web engine search for complicated tasks or frustrating software error messages. Alvin learned to troubleshoot most spreadsheet errors through a web engine search of the error. Chances are high that you if are encountering a problem with some software, someone else has encountered the same problem and has posted a solution on the Internet. We're not saying that tackling all these organizational strategies or technology challenges will be accomplished overnight, but you *can* achieve a healthy level of organization that will help you keep your sanity. Good luck!

Questions for Reflection/Discussion

1. What tools do you have to stay organized?

2. Based on what you need to track, what tools make the most sense for you to use?

3. Does your record-keeping align with your organization's record retention policies?

KEY TAKEAWAYS

- *Keeping your work-related tasks and responsibilities organized is invaluable in performing your job duties because it will save you much-needed time and energy.*

- *Even if orientation is your primary responsibility, all nurse leaders will be charged with managing large amounts of information and other smaller tasks (e.g., budgets). Staying organized is the key to making sure everything is accomplished.*

- *There are many ways to stay organized, so don't be afraid to try something different or talk to others who have a "best practice."*

- *Many resources exist to help you navigate software and applications, so explore these and don't give up!*

Appendix

Essential Orientation Materials for Your Office

You may or may not have a physical office space, but regardless of where you manage your orientation activities, we would like to recommend a few resources for you to keep on hand. Except for the two books written by Alvin, we would like to disclose that we have no personal or financial benefit in recommending these particular resources—they're simply what we use and enjoy.

Books

- This book, the *Staff Educator's Guide to Clinical Orientation* (obviously!): It will get you up and running while hopefully providing you with a concise overview of all activities related to orientation and onboarding.

- The next book in this series, the *Staff Educator's Guide to Professional Development: Assessing and Enhancing Nurse Competency* (Alvin D. Jeffery, M. Anne Longo, & Angela Nienaber, 2015, Sigma Theta Tau International)—Building upon many of these concepts you've already read here, this book focuses on all of the ongoing professional development activities in which an educator would be involved (e.g., inservices).

▓ *Mastering Precepting: A Nurse's Handbook for Success* (Beth Ulrich, 2011, Sigma Theta Tau International)—Preceptors spend more time with orientees than any other stakeholder, so their contributions are invaluable. This book will guide you and them on the path to excellent precepting.

▓ *The Ultimate Guide to Competency Assessment in Health Care* (Donna Wright, 2005, Creative Healthcare Management)—Although Wright's book has a large focus on ongoing competency assessment, many of her principles apply to initial competency assessment, too. She takes a very different approach to this difficult task by making the process extremely practical.

▓ *Nursing Professional Development: Scope and Standards of Practice* (2016, American Nurses Association)—This is a must-have for all nursing professional development specialists. Just like any other nursing specialty, nursing professional development has a scope and standards of practice. This text is the authoritative source of that information.

▓ *The New Mager Six-Pack* (Robert Mager, 1997, Center for Effective Performance)—Mager is the grandfather of modern instructional design. Although the six-pack might seem like overkill at first, this is a great go-to series of books for anyone who is serious about being a great adult educator and instructional designer.

▓ *The Accelerated Learning Fieldbook: Making the Instructional Process Fast, Flexible, and Fun* (Lou Russell, 1999, Pfeiffer)—Russell's book will help you design and develop training more quickly, without sacrificing the rigor. Her book includes a CD-ROM with worksheets, etc.

▓ *Great Webinars: How to Create Interactive Learning That is Captivating, Informative, and Fun* (Cynthia Clay, 2012, Pfeiffer)—Clay teaches seminars based on her book and really helps bring webinars to life. She shows the reader how to with great, practical examples. She reminds us to keep the learners front and center as we build webinars.

▓ *Creative New Employee Orientation Programs: Best Practices, Creative Ideas, and Activities for Energizing Your Orientation Program* (Doris M. Sims, 2002, McGraw-Hill)—The author provides best practices and lots and lots of checklists for your use. Her approach is focused more at the organizational level, but many of the checklists could be adapted for use at a unit level. This one is an oldie, but a goodie!

■ *Developing a Residency in Post-Acute Care* (Edna Cadmus et al., 2017, Sigma Theta Tau International)—The authors provide a very in-depth and holistic approach to developing a residency program. Primarily focused on geriatric, post-acute care, this exhaustive reference can easily be adapted for any healthcare setting.

Websites

■ http://www.thiagi.com—Dr. Sivasailam Thiagarajan (Thiagi) started his business almost 40 years ago and his mission remains the same: "to help people achieve more through performance-based training that is motivating and effective." Thiagi is a great resource for games and other low-tech approaches to help groups learn information quickly and in a fun environment. He has many free downloads available on his site.

■ http://www.trainerswarehouse.com—Trainers Warehouse provides items that you can use for (primarily) classroom-based activities. Want to set up your own version of *Jeopardy!* to facilitate learning a certain topic? Trainers Warehouse can help. Have a long classroom session and want some basic toys on the table to keep your adult learners occupied? They've got that kind of stuff, too!

■ http://www.instructionaldesigncentral.com—Instructional Design Central is a website that provides resources and information for instructional designers.

Stay up-to-date with your nursing journals and websites as well, and look for websites that focus specifically on being a professional development specialist in nursing! Here are some websites to get you started:

■ http://www.anpd.org—Association for Nursing Professional Development

■ http://pneg.org/—Professional Nurse Educators Group

■ http://journals.lww.com/jnsdonline—*Journal for Nurses in Professional Development*

■ http://www.nursecredentialing.org/ NursingProfessionalDevelopment—Certification resources

1-Minute Literature Review

Even though books are great resources for developing or enhancing onboarding programs, there is also merit in having peer-reviewed articles available. Especially in organizations that have a large emphasis on evidence-based decision-making, you may be asked for "proof" that a particular change is warranted. Therefore, we want to provide you with several articles we believe are beneficial for you to have on hand. Due to the rapid nature with which new articles are published, this list may quickly become dated, but if you're short on time, this is a good place to start.

General Orientation/Onboarding Literature

Title: The Effectiveness of an Organizational-Level Orientation Training Program in Socialization of New Hires

Year/Author: 2000; Howard J. Klein & Natasha A. Weaver

Journal/Volume/Issue/Page: *Personnel Psychology, 53*(1), 47–66

Description: The authors look at the impact of organizational-level orientation in over 100 employees in different disciplines and industries before and at the 1- and 2-month marks. They found that employees who participated in an organizational-level orientation were more likely to be socialized about the goals and mission of the organization, as well as its history and people.

Title: Onboarding New Employees: Maximizing Success

Year/Author: 2010; Talya N. Bauer

Journal/Volume/Issue/Page: *SHRM Foundation Effective Practice Guideline Series*, 1–54

Description: Dr. Bauer addresses different (effective) approaches for onboarding new employees. She also explores short- and long-term outcomes that should be part of an effective onboarding program. Her Four C's model is included in Chapter 2 of this book.

Title: New-Hire Onboarding: Common Mistakes to Avoid

Year/Author: 2013; Alexia Vernon

Journal/Volume/Issue/Page: *T&D, 66(9),* 32–33

Description: This short article addresses five key mistakes to avoid when onboarding, especially when onboarding new college graduates. The author discusses strategies for avoiding these common mistakes, as well as the importance of engaging your new employees on day one.

Nursing-Specific Literature

Title: Nurses' Hospital Orientation and Future Research Challenges: An Integrative Review

Year/Author: 2016; J. Peltokoski, K. Vehvilainen-Julkunen, & M. Miettinen

Journal/Volume/Issue/Page: *International Nursing Review, 63,* 92–103

Description: The number of research studies that identify and explore best orientation practices are very limited. This literature review includes 11 such research studies that focus on hospital-based nursing orientation programs. Many of these practices will not be new to you, and we've discussed most of them in this book. However, this is a great article to keep on hand if you're looking for research that would help you decide whether to adopt certain orientation and onboarding practices.

Title: A Magnetic Strategy for New Graduate Nurses

Year/Author: 2007; Diana Halfer

Journal/Volume/Issue/Page: *Nursing Economic$, 25(1),* 6–11

Description: This article describes one hospital's major overhaul of their orientation program, which reduced new graduate RN turnover from 29.5% to 12.3%. They developed a holistic orientation/onboarding program that involved classroom training (general and specialty content along with advanced life support), structured mentorship, preceptor development, professional transition support, and debriefings.

Title: Specialized New Graduate RN Pediatric Orientation: A Strategy for Nursing Retention and Its Financial Impact

Year/Author: 2013; M. Isabel Friedman, Margaret M. Delaney, Kathleen Schmidt, Carolyn Quinn, & Irene Macyk

Journal/Volume/Issue/Page: *Nursing Economic$, 31*(4), 162–170

Description: In addition to demonstrating the financial impact of a well-developed onboarding program, this article contains several tables with content and timeline details of a year-long fellowship program for new graduate RNs entering specialty fields (critical care, emergency department, and hematology/oncology).

Title: New Graduate Nurse Residency: A Network Approach

Year/Author: 2013; Jeanette P. Little, Dianne Ditmer, & Marie A. Bashaw

Journal/Volume/Issue/Page: *Journal of Nursing Administration, 43*(6), 361–366

Description: This article describes a multi-site organization's approach to creating a new residency program and provides several details on the content and structure. A really nice feature of this article is the authors' inclusion of their outcome measures for evaluating the program and some financial information that you might be able to use to calculate your own ROI.

Title: Orientation to Emergency Nursing: Perceptions of New Graduate Nurses

Year/Author: 2010; Barbara Patterson, Elizabeth W. Bayley, Krista Burnell, & Jan Rhoads

Journal/Volume/Issue/Page: *Journal of Emergency Nursing, 36*(3), 203–211

Description: This research study used qualitative and quantitative methods to discover strengths as well as improvement opportunities for a 6-month fellowship program for new graduate RNs working in an emergency department. Strengths included length of program, support from key stakeholders, interpersonal relationship development within a cohort, and variety of learning materials and classes. Opportunities for improvement included dispersing class sessions throughout the program (rather than at the beginning), focusing classroom content on specialty, increasing the use of simulation (and other interactive activities), and providing more debriefing and discussion opportunities.

Title: Newly Graduated Nurses' Orientation Experiences: A Systematic Review of Qualitative Studies

Year/Author: 2017; Katariina Pasila, Satu Elo, & Maria Kaariainen

Journal/Volume/Issue/Page: *International Journal of Nursing Studies, 71,* 17–27

Description: If you're looking for insights into new graduate nurses' perceptions and experiences with a wide variety of programs, this review article will be very helpful. The authors integrated findings from 13 qualitative research studies to develop new themes to describe experiences.

Title: Solving the Retention Puzzle: Let's Begin with Nursing Orientation

Year/Author: 2012; Betsy Brakovich & Elizabeth Bonham

Journal/Volume/Issue/Page: *Nurse Leader, 10(5),* 50–53, 61

Description: The authors of this article used the Casey-Fink Graduate Nurse Experience Survey to explore the perceptions of new graduate RNs during their third month of employment. They describe the perspective of four different cohorts in the areas of skill and procedure performance, confidence and stressors, role transition, confidence and critical-thinking skills, time management, role responsibility, communication, and support in the work environment. This article provides a summary of what many new graduate RNs are thinking at the 3-month mark.

Title: An Interdepartmental Team Approach to Develop, Implement, and Sustain an Oncology Nursing Orientation Program

Year/Author: 2011; Nancy Kuhrik, Linda Laub, Marilee Kuhrik, & Kathy Atwater

Journal/Volume/Issue/Page: *Oncology Nursing Forum, 38(2),* 115–118

Description: These authors provide the reader with specific outlines and objectives of their orientation schedule. Although the content is specific to oncology nursing, their format could be easily adapted to your individual needs.

Title: Progress Meetings: Facilitating Role Transition of the New Graduate Nurse

Year/Author: 2009; Marlene Goodwin-Esola, Maureen Deely, & Nancy Powell

Journal/Volume/Issue/Page: *The Journal of Continuing Education in Nursing, 40*(9), 411–415

Description: This article details a practical method for meeting regularly with new graduate RNs to assess their progress and help them transition into their new roles. By meeting regularly and consistently to assess competency development, the new nurse not only transitions more smoothly, but also develops stronger relationships with the managers and educators.

Title: Job Integration Factors as Predictors of Travel Nurse Job Performance: A Mixed-Methods Study

Year/Author: 2015; Carol A. Tuttas

Journal/Volume/Issue/Page: *Journal of Nursing Care Quality, 30*(1), 44–52

Description: This article describes a research study with focus-group interviews and a quantitative survey of travel nurses. The qualitative findings of traveler preferences for orientation and onboarding are particularly relevant for staff educators. A few key points include providing pre-assignment instructions on where and when to be on Day 1, streamlining orientation content that may be similar between organizations (e.g., hand washing), facilitating communication with staff and leadership, focusing on unit-specific policies and workflows, and serving as an "ambassador" for questions that may arise during the assignment.

INDEX